It's Not You,

It's Cancer

~~~~~~~~~~~~~~~~~~~~~~~~~~~~~

A Slightly Inappropriate Guide to
Breast Cancer Survival

~~~~~~~~~~~~~~~

Author: Brenda M. Lee

This book is intended for informational and educational purposes only. It is not a substitute for professional medical advice, diagnosis, or treatment. Always consult your physician or other qualified healthcare provider with any questions you may have regarding a medical condition.

While every effort has been made to ensure the accuracy of the information at the time of publication, medical understanding continues to evolve. Readers are encouraged to keep learning and to work closely with their healthcare teams.

This book was made possible through the stories, support, and strength of survivors everywhere. You are seen. You are valued. You are not alone.

For permissions, inquiries, or speaking opportunities, contact:
BLeePhotog@gmail.com | **brendamlee.wordpress.com**

First Edition, 2025
Printed in the United States of America

ISBN: 979-8-9937220-0-9
Cover and Interior Design by Brenda M. Lee
Author photo by JWLee Media, LLC

📖 Table of Contents

Dedication

To my Aunt Linda, diagnosed at 29 and still raising hell decades later. I was just a kid when you faced cancer, but your story always lived in the back of my mind like a quiet kind of hope. You were proof that survival was possible long before I needed that proof for myself. You've always been my hero—not just for beating cancer, but for the way you carry strength with grace and grit. Thank you for blazing the trail.

To my bestie, Jessica—my ride-or-die, "no judgment" zone. You never question my sanity (even when you probably should). You show up for the raw, the ugly, the weird, and the tequila-fueled. You've talked me down, lifted me up, and made me laugh through more tears than I can count. There's comfort in knowing I can say literally anything, and your response will be, "Yeah, that tracks."

To my kids—Ashleigh, Carley, Lauryn, and Jackson. Watching you grow has been the greatest joy of my life, and being here for you is the role I cherish most. You've taught me patience (well... sort of), resilience, and how to find light even in the hardest seasons. I hope I've made you proud. You've certainly made me proud—gray hair and all.

To my mom, Gloria. Our personalities didn't always match, and we had our battles. But one thing I never doubted was that you had my back when it counted. You were one phone call away, always ready with a pep talk that was equal parts love and "get your shit together." I miss that. I miss you. I hope you'd be proud of this book—and of me.

To my husband, Jonathan. You are the calm in my chaos. You've never once rolled your eyes at my endless new projects, my shifting dreams, or the half-finished ideas I scatter like confetti. You believe in me more than I believe in myself sometimes, and your steady presence lets me take chances I might otherwise run from. This time, I followed through. Because you never stopped cheering.

And to Tammy. You were there when my world was falling apart. You kept my kids safe, my fridge full, and my head above water. I wish I could have been better for you when you needed me. I didn't—and I've carried that. Your friendship taught me what it means to really show up for someone. I'm still learning. Still trying. You left a mark I won't forget.

"She stood in the storm, and when the wind did not blow her way, she adjusted her sails."
—Elizabeth Edwards

Dear Reader,

If you're holding this book, chances are you, or someone you love, recently heard the words, "You have breast cancer."

Your world feels wide open and raw. You're probably terrified about all of the unknowns. Or, if you're like I was, you're currently totally numb. Maybe you're angry, confused, in denial, or stuck in that in-between space where you're just waiting for someone to tell you what the heck to do next.

Wherever you are in this mess of a journey, beginning, middle, or end, please hear me:
You do not have to do this alone.

This path can be a whole lot less brutal if you surround yourself with people who get it. People who don't flinch when you talk about drains or dead nipples or the breakdown you had while hiding in your car after your fourth appointment of the day. Surround yourself with people that nod and say, "Yep. I've done that too," because chances are that whatever you're feeling is perfectly normal, and someone else has felt exactly the same way.

You're going to need real connection. Real people with real voices and real, relatable stories.
That's what this book is for. A way to find connection in a massive world that feels like it's spinning way too fast.

When I got the Cancer Phone Call all those years ago, my brain just… flatlined. Shock doesn't even begin to cover it. My mind went numb, my ears were ringing, and it felt like I was underwater. Doctors were using words that went way over my head, and I was suddenly drowning in medical jargon that I didn't understand, and being asked to make decisions I didn't feel capable of making. People were talking at me, but it all sounded like background noise. I couldn't focus. I couldn't think. I couldn't even ask the right questions, because I was so overwhelmed and didn't know where to begin, or what the hell was happening. So I just nodded along and did what I was told.

Ultimately, that was why I decided to write this book. I wish I'd had a guide like this to help me. Someone that has "been there" to

9

figuratively hold my hand and help me be better educated in the decisions I would need to make. Someone to guide me along and show me different paths. Google can be way too much, but we all need a safe place to start.

Let me back up for a second. Just so we're clear, I'm not some expert in a white coat. I'm not a surgeon, an oncologist, or a cancer researcher. I don't have a fancy degree hanging on my wall. I haven't been to school for any of this. I'm writing about my experience and those that I interviewed. I don't have all the answers, but hopefully this book can help you feel more seen, and give you a starting point on choices to make and questions to ask.

So what qualifies me to write a book about breast cancer? Why should you bother to read my book instead of one written by a doctor? Because what I *do* have is experience. A survivor's perspective, and the ability to share what I've been through. And as you're about to find out, I've been through some shit, believe me. I don't claim to have all the answers, but I've had the rug yanked out from under my life and stared heartbreak and fear right in the face. I've broken down and cried with strangers in waiting rooms. I've shared dark humor with other warriors while chemo dripped into my veins. I coped poorly, I drank too much alcohol and smoked too many cigarettes all in an effort to just find some peace. I also divorced my husband, and lost my best friend. But that's just me. If you look up "shitshow" in the dictionary, there I am. A photo of me, in all my bald glory. Not everyone goes through the same experiences I did. In fact, a lot of people become closer to families and friends. We all have our own stories to write, and I'll be sharing some of them here.

So, in a nutshell, after what was the hardest year of my life, here's what I do know:

Cancer is absolute bullshit. Full stop. There's no getting around it. But damn, if it doesn't teach you a lot about who you are, and the people you surround yourself with.

Today, I'm healthy. I'm alive. I've even donated a kidney for a family member, 6 weeks before my 50th birthday. I'm a hell of a lot stronger than I was when this all started.

I finished treatment in 2008, and it's taken me this long to write this book because, truth be told, it took that long for me to make peace with everything. In this book, I'll talk about my trauma. The rage. The way cancer forced me to rebuild everything from the ground up. There's no timeline on healing, and I am a stubborn, hard-headed woman. I found the longest road possible, and still dragged my feet the whole time. Your girl can really hold a grudge!

But I'm here now, for you, to share with you my journey, in hopes that I can help you navigate the choices that I had to make without anybody's help.

I'm writing this for you so you don't have to feel as lost as I did. If my experiences (and screw-ups) can help light the way, even a little, then every ugly, painful, beautiful, messy part of this will have been worth it.

This book shares my story, and the stories of others, as we stumbled, swore, cried, and clawed our way through our cancer seasons. Your path won't look exactly like ours. But maybe—just maybe—you'll relate to something we talk about in here, and some of these stories will make you feel seen. Make you nod, saying, "Me too."

In the end, I want to give you something solid to hold on to. I'm here to share in the hope for what's ahead. I'm a little snarky, and very blunt, so if you're not careful, I might even get you to smile once in a while.

I'm not here to play doctor. I'm not qualified to give you medical advice, and although this book might not cover every single thing ever presented, it will give you a baseline to start conversations with your cancer team. I will tell you what your options are, so you know what kind of research to start with and how to figure out what's best for your body. I'll show you how to ask better questions, and how to advocate for yourself. We'll talk about how to protect your sanity, and how to care for the people you love without losing yourself in the process. I even included a resource section in the back for when your Google-machine just isn't cutting it anymore.

More than anything, I want you to feel less alone while you're walking through this, because cancer is a very lonely place. Finding people with the same experiences as you will make it feel a lot less lonely.

There will be fear and there will be doubt.

People will surprise you, disappoint you, and show up in ways you never could have guessed.
Above all, there will also be healing.
And I'll be right here, walking with you, one step at a time.

With all my love,
Brenda M. Lee

1

The Quiet Voice that Saves You

There was a time when my life felt wide open and full of light. I was married, living in Sunny Florida, raising two daughters, and a scruffy little dog named Dee-Oh-Jee. Our circle of friends was close. They were the kind of group that didn't need an invitation to stop by. Weekends often meant BBQs that stretched long past sunset, with the adults sipping drinks and talking about everything and nothing, while the kids raced around with bare feet, sticky fingers, and the kind of wild imagination that only comes from childhood summers. Bikes lay scattered in the driveway. Sleeping bags took over living room floors. It was the warm, noisy rhythm that makes you believe life is good and nothing could ever ruin it.

At thirty years old, my days were full. Mornings meant brushing ponytails, packing lunches, folding laundry, and running errands. Afternoons sometimes found me riding on the back of my husband's motorcycle, wind tangling my hair, before racing back for school pickup, homework, and the evening scramble toward dinner. Our marriage had its cracks, but I wasn't worried. What marriage is perfect? We were messy and normal, and I thought that was enough.

I'd heard about self-breast exams; seen the pamphlets in waiting rooms, and probably heard them mentioned in high school health class, but I didn't do them. I felt fine. Young. Strong. Untouchable. Cancer was something that happened to other people, far away from my little world.

Then one routine appointment changed everything.

I didn't feel that tiny lump at the top of my right breast, my gynecologist did. I had no symptoms. No warning signs. No reason to think anything could be wrong. But she noticed what I didn't. To this day, I still wonder what might have happened if I'd skipped that checkup. If I'd let laundry, errands, or groceries matter more than a fifteen-minute appointment. How long would it have taken me to find it that lump? Would I have been too late?

Now pause for a moment and think about eight women you know: friends, family, coworkers. Picture their faces. Hear their voices. And if you're a woman, count yourself among them. **One in eight will be diagnosed with breast cancer.**That's not an exaggerated statistic meant to scare you. It's reality. Breast cancer is the most common cancer in women worldwide, and while treatments have come a long way, more than 40,000 women still die every year in the U.S. alone.

It's not just older women, either. Breast cancer is showing up earlier and earlier than it used to. In the past decade, cases in women under 40 have risen by more than two percent every year. That might sound small until it's you, or someone you love, becoming part of that number. I was 31 years old when I was diagnosed with Invasive Ductal Carcinoma.

Around the early 2000's, mammogram guidelines were all over the place. Some said start at 50, others said 40, and it felt like no one agreed. Thankfully, most major medical groups now recommend routine mammograms beginning at age 40 for women at average risk. That shift came about because breast cancer in women under 50 years old has been climbing, and early detection can save lives.

Family history can change this picture entirely. I was 31 when diagnosed. My aunt was only 29. There's no genetic marker waving a red flag in our bloodwork, but cancer clearly runs in our family. That's why my daughter learned about self-breast exams early and began yearly mammograms at 23. She's seen firsthand what happens when cancer sneaks in quietly, and she wants to be ready. I support that with my whole heart.

If you have a family history like ours, or even if something just doesn't feel right, talk to your doctor. You don't need to wait for permission or follow a one-size-fits-all guideline. **Your intuition matters.** You're allowed to say, "I want to be checked."

So, if you're not doing monthly self-breast exams, please start. If you have daughters, teach them. Talk to them about why it matters. Make sure they know their bodies so they'll notice when something changes. This doesn't just happen to "other people." It can happen to anyone, no matter how healthy or happy you feel. Cancer doesn't wait for life to slow down.

That's one of the reasons I wrote this book. There were so many things I wish I'd known. I wasn't prepared. I thought it didn't apply to me. I had no idea what to do after hearing those three words: **"You have cancer."**

I was never handed a treasure map to guide me through. No instruction manual to tell me what came next. Just a terrifying, confusing blur where everything I knew shifted in an instant. This book isn't a cure, but maybe it can be a flashlight. A little light in the dark to help you take the next step when the ground feels unsteady.

One thing I've learned is that the person you were before your diagnosis is gone. You are forever changed. This path you're about to walk will be different and harder than anything you've done before. The way you think, the way you see the world, how you treat your body, and even the way you interact with family will shift, sometimes in ways you can't predict. Cancer leaves its mark on everything. And you get to choose whether it changes you for the better or pulls you under. In my case, I let it pull me under for a while, and I wouldn't recommend that to anyone.

The most important thing right now is learning how to navigate this system and advocate for yourself, for the best outcome both physically and emotionally. It starts with trusting your intuition. If something feels wrong, keep pushing for answers, even if a doctor brushes it off.

Joyce's Story – Trusting Her Gut

I didn't find my own lump, mostly because I wasn't doing monthly self-exams like I should have been. My friend, Joyce, had the opposite experience.

Her story began in October of 1999. She was 43 years old, had no family history of breast cancer, and had recently had a mammogram that came back clear. On paper, everything looked perfectly normal.

Then one evening, while watching television, Joyce happened across a program about breast cancer and the importance of self-exams. She wasn't worried—she had small breasts, hadn't noticed any changes, and wasn't feeling any pain. But something in her gut told her to check anyway.

15

That instinct saved her life.

What she felt stopped her cold. Her entire left breast, from the chest wall to the nipple and wrapping around both sides, was hard. Not a small bump, but a solid mass about the size of her palm. She knew instantly that something was wrong. Later, her doctors confirmed what her instincts had already told her—that chance moment in front of the TV had changed everything.

Joyce's experience was the opposite of mine in nearly every way. When I shut down after hearing the news, she stayed grounded. Where I panicked, she prayed. Where I questioned everything, she trusted a path she couldn't yet see.

Her strength didn't come from having all the answers—it came from an unshakable faith that no matter what happened, she wouldn't be facing it alone. While I struggled to get my bearings, Joyce leaned on her family, her church, and her God. Her voice carries a calmness when she speaks, full of grace and conviction.

Though our stories are different, her courage and peace in the face of fear are qualities I deeply respect.

💔 Faith, Anger, and Silence

I wish I could tell you that my faith held steady to get me through my cancer diagnosis; that I found comfort in prayer or leaned into God when I couldn't sleep at night. But that wasn't my story.

The truth is, God and I didn't speak for a long time. I was angry; deep down, bone-deep angry. I felt abandoned, punished for something I didn't do. And if I had nothing nice to say, I said nothing at all. That silence lasted years. Fifteen, to be exact.

It took a long time to return to anything that felt like faith. Even now, my faith doesn't look the way it once did. I'm still piecing it together.

Andrea's story echoes a similar ache. She told me:

"I was angry. Angry at the world. Angry at the cancer. Angry at God. I didn't understand how something so cruel could happen and still

16

believe in a God that was good. I had to let go of everything I thought I knew and start over from the bottom."

I knew exactly what she meant. You think you believe. You are firm in your faith, until something tears through your life and leaves you holding the pieces. The journey back, if there is one, isn't straight. Sometimes it doesn't take you back at all. Sometimes it leads you somewhere entirely new.

There's no single way to heal spiritually. Some people find strength in scripture, others in nature, therapy, meditation, or simply surviving the day in front of them. But I've noticed something in talking with different survivors: those who managed to hold on to their faith, in whatever form it took, often walked away from their cancer experience with less bitterness and less confusion. Those who, like me, turned away for a time tended to carry the weight of it for much longer.

If your faith feels broken, or gone altogether, know this: you are not alone. You're allowed to question. You're allowed to be angry. And you're allowed to take your time finding whatever peace looks like for you. But if you're able to come back around and find it again, I've seen it help so many people get through the hardest journey of their lives.

Why Listening Matters

That's the thing about cancer. You really have to pay attention to the smallest whispers from your body.

Doctors are highly trained, but they're still human. And humans make mistakes. Misdiagnoses happen. Patients get brushed off.

Too many young women are told it's "probably nothing," that they're "too young" for breast cancer, or that they should *just wait and see.* Those words have cost people their lives.

I'm grateful every single day that my doctor didn't dismiss the small lump she found just because I was thirty. She didn't tell me I was wasting her time. She trusted her instincts, and I believe that decision saved my life.

17

If something feels wrong, speak up. If no one's listening, speak louder. And if they still won't listen, find someone who will. **Your voice matters in that exam room.** Asking questions is your right, and so is getting a second or even third opinion.

"Early detection saves lives" isn't just a slogan. The earlier cancer is caught, the more treatment options you have. Those treatments may be less aggressive, and your chances of survival are much higher.

In the end, even if your concerns turn out to be nothing, that's okay! You'll walk away with something far too many people fighting this disease wish they could have: peace of mind.

✂ Practical Tips: How to Listen to Your Body

- Do a self-breast exam monthly, ideally a few days after your period, or on the same day each month if you don't menstruate. Learn how to do an exam properly at nationalbreastcancer.org/breast-self-exam.

- Keep a notes app on your phone where you can record symptoms or questions between visits.

- Don't wait for your annual checkup. If something feels wrong, call and ask to be seen.

- Be clear when calling. Tell them it's about a breast concern and ask if there's a nurse you can talk to.

✒ Karol Ann M. – Diagnosed at 39 & 40

Sometimes, listening to your body means doing the thing you least want to do: going back for another scan.

Karol Ann was 39 the first time early detection saved her life. An MRI picked up a suspicious spot, and a biopsy confirmed what nobody wants to hear: Stage 1 invasive ductal carcinoma. Triple positive.

The doctor told her over a FaceTime call. She says she can remember the faint pixelation on the screen, the tinny sound of the doctor's voice, and the way the world seemed to go suddenly quiet. Her hands went cold and her stomach tightened. Karol Ann said she was suddenly angry. And scared. It felt like she was slipping out of her own body, watching the moment happen from somewhere far above.

Treatment began immediately. Two lumpectomies, chemotherapy, immunotherapy, radiation, and hormone blockers. Karol Ann followed every instruction to the letter. She showed up for every scan and appointment. She sat in cold exam rooms under fluorescent lights, pretending she wasn't terrified.

When treatment ended, she said she let herself believe, just for a while, that she was done.

A year later, that illusion shattered. Karol Ann's first post-treatment mammogram brought the words she had feared: *new calcifications*. Another biopsy. The antiseptic smell of the imaging room and the technician's silence told her the truth before the results even came back. Her gut already knew.

This time, it was invasive lobular carcinoma in the opposite breast. Another wave of impossible choices. This time, she chose a double mastectomy. After everything she had already been through, she just couldn't sit and wait for another blow. Karol Ann needed to feel in control again.

If she had ignored those follow-up scans, she might not be here to share her story. That second diagnosis was caught early enough for the doctors to act fast.

Her advice to anyone reading this: **never skip your scans.** Not when you're scared. Not when you feel fine. Not when you think you've already survived the worst. Twice now, early detection has saved her life.

Questions to Reflect On

- Have I noticed any recent physical or emotional changes I've ignored?

- When was the last time I did a self-breast exam or requested one?

- Is there a part of my care plan I don't fully understand but have hesitated to question?

- Who is the medical professional I trust most, and why?

Chapter Highlights

- Monthly self-breast exams are a critical tool for early detection.

- Early detection significantly increases treatment options and survival rates.

- Trusting your gut and advocating for yourself can save your life.

- Tracking physical and emotional changes can help prepare for appointments.

Key Takeaway

Learning to trust your body and your instincts can be crucial when it comes to advocating for yourself. This is not an overreaction—you are worth the time and attention it takes to listen, notice, and speak up.

"The key to life is accepting challenges. Once someone stops doing this, he's dead."
—Bette Davis, on resilience and not letting illness define you.

2
It's Probably Nothing...

Early detection saved my life.

There I was, sitting in the patient exam room at my routine ladies' appointment. The paper gown crinkled and itched against my skin, and the air in the room was cool enough to give me goosebumps. My feet dangled above the floor until the doctor pulled the footrest out and asked me to lie back.

Her gloved fingers began their familiar path, moving with practiced precision across my skin. I stared at the ceiling tiles, counting them without really keeping track, my mind drifting toward dinner plans and whether I'd have time to swing by the grocery store before the girls got out of school.

Then her hand paused. Just for a moment, but it was enough to pull me straight out of my daydream. My eyes went from the ceiling to her face, searching for something to tell me it was nothing. Her expression barely changed, but I caught it: the slight furrow in her brow, the smallest downturn of her lip, the breath she took that lasted just a second longer than it should have.

She took my hand and guided my fingers to what she had found: a small lump high on the upper part of my right breast.

"I'd like to send you for a mammogram today," she said, helping me sit up. Her voice was steady, but there was something in it that told me this was important.

I nodded, even tried to smile, feeling the first thread of annoyance about how much time this was going to take. Should I call my husband to pick up the girls? Could I still get to the grocery store? I brushed at the tingle running up the back of my neck, but something inside me had shifted. My chest felt tight, my heart beating faster than it should. I realized I'd been holding my breath without meaning to. I told myself I was being dramatic. I was young. I was healthy. This wasn't going to be anything serious.

Still, a flicker of doubt stayed lodged just beneath the surface.

The mammogram machine was cold, the metal plates hard against my skin. When they pressed together, it felt like the air was being squeezed out of my lungs. I stared ahead, willing myself not to flinch, trying to keep my thoughts away from my aunt who had been diagnosed with breast cancer at 29, just a year younger than I was then.

Relief came quickly. The radiologist glanced at the images, offered a polite smile, and said, "Probably just a cyst. Your body will most likely absorb it naturally. Come back in six months and we'll take another look."

As I walked back to my car in the heavy Florida heat, I exhaled. My shoulders dropped. I even laughed a little at myself for letting worry take up so much space in my head. But months later, that worry would come back. And this time, it would be anything but silly.

✎ Maggie G.

"I was 50 years old when I went in for my routine mammogram. I wasn't worried. I had no pain, no symptoms. When they called me back for a follow-up, I still wasn't that worried. They said it was probably just dense tissue. Even when I went in for a biopsy, I told myself, 'It's just a precaution.' I didn't mention it to my kids or even my husband. I thought I'd save them the worry. When the call finally came, I was at work. I took it in the stairwell so no one would hear. I remember sliding down the wall, my back against the railing, just trying to breathe."

These kinds of stories are ones that so many people can relate to. That strange cocktail of reassurance and dread. It's the mind's way of trying to protect the heart. You hope and pray. You rationalize. You carry on. Until suddenly, you can't anymore.

▦ What to Expect at Your First Imaging

- Compression is uncomfortable, but necessary to get clear images.

- Waiting for results is often the most stressful part. Try to remember that many findings are benign. Ask your doctor to order a "Diagnostic Mammogram" if you can't wait. They should give you the results before you leave the office.

- More imaging may be needed. If your doctor sees something they want to get a better look at, you might be sent for an ultrasound or MRI. I know it sounds scary, but try not to panic. These extra steps help your doctor give you the best care possible when they can't see due to dense tissue, and very often, there's nothing serious behind them.

✎ Julie P.

"My doctor almost didn't send me for a mammogram. I had just turned 40 and went in for my annual physical. I didn't have a lump, and no obvious symptoms. Just a gut feeling that something wasn't right. My doctor said it was probably nothing. But I pushed. I insisted, and that mammogram saved my life. They found a 1.2 cm tumor, DCIS, and it was already starting to spread. I think about it all the time, how easy it would've been to just nod, agree, and walk out of her office without getting tested. If I hadn't spoken up, and pushed for the mammogram, I might not be here today."

Julie's story is a quiet but powerful reminder: **your intuition matters.**

Even if it feels awkward or if you feel like you're being "pushy." **Speak up.** Ask for the test. Ask again and again if you have to.

You know your body better than anyone, and sometimes, that small voice inside you is just trying to save your life. You have to be your own advocate.

✎ Thermography: A Secondary Option for Those Who Can't Tolerate Mammograms

Some people find the compression of a mammogram physically unbearable. Others may have medical conditions that make even low-doses of radiation feel like a risk. For them, infrared thermography is sometimes considered as an alternative. Unlike traditional mammograms that use X-rays, thermography involves sitting in front of a camera that reads the heat patterns in and just below your skin. There's no squeezing, no paddles, and no radiation.

But, thermography comes with some serious limitations. While a mammogram can detect the tiniest signs of cancer before you can even feel a lump, thermography can only pick up changes in temperature. These "hot spots" might signal something unusual, but they can also be caused by non-cancerous things like inflammation, infection, or even something as simple as a tight sports bra. **That's why thermography is not considered reliable for detecting early-stage breast cancer.** Many hospitals don't offer it, and insurance companies are often hesitant to cover it because it's not held to the same rigorous standards as mammography.

In short, thermography may be helpful for those who truly can't undergo a mammogram, but it's not a substitute. If it's the only option you have right now, it's better than nothing. But the goal should always be to return to standard screening as soon as it's safe and possible to do so.

What's a BI-RADS Score?

If your imaging results include something called a **BI-RADS score**, you may be wondering what that means. It's a number your radiologist uses to describe what they see on your mammogram or ultrasound. The scale runs from **0 to 6**, and each number helps guide your next steps. A lower number usually means everything looks normal, while a higher number means more follow-up is needed, or a biopsy might be warranted. It's a way for doctors to stay consistent in how they report findings, and it's a helpful tool that you and your medical team can use to make informed decisions together.

Erica L.

"When I first felt the lump, it felt like a marble under my skin. I figured it was a clogged duct, or maybe a cyst. Nothing urgent. I didn't have insurance at the time, so I waited. I waited six months. By the time I saw a doctor, everything moved fast; imaging, biopsy, diagnosis. I was 33. No family history. Still, it was cancer. Stage 2B. I'll always wonder how things might've been different if I'd gone in sooner. But I also know how easy it is to hope something will just... go away."

Erica's honesty is painfully common.
As women, so many of us put ourselves last. We worry about everything and everyone ahead of ourselves. Finances. Family. Fear. It all piles up and whispers, *"Just wait a little longer."*

If no one else has said it, let me:
If something feels off, you are worth the follow-up.
You're worth the appointment.
You're worth the cost.
You're worth the time.

✎ Rena W.

"I was so nervous during the biopsy that I nearly passed out. Not from pain. It really wasn't painful. But the panic was unreal. I felt like I couldn't breathe, like I was floating outside my body. The doctor and nurse were kind, but the whole thing felt cold. Clinical. Mechanical. I wish someone had told me I could ask for something to help with the anxiety. It wasn't until I joined a support group that I found out that's an option."

Rena's story shines a light on something so many women never hear until it's too late: **you're allowed to ask for help, especially when it's "just" emotional.**

Procedures can be triggering. They can awaken trauma or leave you spiraling inside your own head. This is such a normal, natural reaction.

If you're scared, it's perfectly normal, and it's okay to say so.
If you need something to calm your nerves, ask for help.
You do not have to be stoic. There's absolutely nothing to prove here.
You deserve to feel safe.

🧠 Questions to Ask Your Doctor

- What did you find during the exam that concerns you?

- Could this be benign? What are other possible explanations?

- How dense is my breast tissue, and does that affect accuracy?

- Should I have additional imaging before the biopsy (like ultrasound or MRI)?

- What type of biopsy do you recommend, and why?

- Will I be awake for the biopsy? Can I request sedation?

- How long will results take, and how will I receive them?

- What side effects (bruising, soreness) should I expect afterward?

- Are there emotional support resources while I wait?

My Biopsy

A week after my second mammogram, I lay on the exam table under the glare of fluorescent lights. The room was warm and quiet, except for the soft clinking of metal instruments being arranged on a tray nearby. I stared up at the ceiling tiles, trying to focus on anything outside of that room, but my thoughts kept drifting to all the things this could mean. All the outcomes I didn't want to say out loud.

When they began the biopsy, I kept glancing down toward my chest, trying to see what they were doing. But their hands were too close to my face, blocking my view. It felt like there were too many people in the room. Too many voices. Too many people touching me. I felt hot and cold and overwhelmed all at once.

I was a lab specimen instead of a human being. My fear was barely held in place.

The needle pierced too close to my heart, both physically and emotionally.

No one had warned me how terrifying this simple procedure would be. It didn't hurt. The numbing agent did its job. But the panic of being laid bare while strangers worked silently over me. *That* was unbearable.

Looking back, I'm still shocked it wasn't standard procedure to offer something to ease my anxiety. No sedative. No preparation. Not even

any words of encouragement.
Just *get on the table, hold still and try not to fall apart.*

But I did fall apart.
The buzzing in my ears. The tightness in my throat. The tears I tried to blink away before anyone noticed. I bit my lip, willing myself to stay still and to be brave. Whatever that meant.

But the tears just came anyway. No matter how much I fought it. No matter how strong I tried to be, they just kept coming. Not from pain, but from everything else. It was all just too much.

I remember the nurse reaching out, gently patting my hand. Her voice was soft, calm, almost a whisper. "It could be nothing," she said. "It's too soon to worry."

But I already knew.
I felt the truth in the back of my mind. It was settled deep in the pit of my stomach. There was no part of me that didn't already know exactly what the answer would be.

Later, on the way home, I sat in the passenger seat of my friend's car, staring out the window while the world passed us by. I didn't see any of it. I don't know what she talked about. It was like I had floated outside of myself, watching the hollow shell of who I used to be.

I had disappeared into nothingness.

Not everyone feels this overwhelmed during their biopsy. Some people take it in stride. I don't know why my mind reacted the way it did, but like a lot of things in high stress situations: until it happens to *you*, you don't know how you'll react.

My advice is to go slow and give yourself permission to breathe.
Find something—*anything*—to distract your mind.
And most importantly?

Ask for the sedative.
If you think you might need it, don't hesitate.
I wish someone had told me that.
Because I sure as hell could've used it.

🔬 Biopsy Basics

Purpose: Confirm whether a suspicious mass is cancerous and identify the tumor type.
Common Types:

- *Core Needle Biopsy:* larger tissue sample

- *Fine Needle Aspiration (FNA):* fluid or cells

- *Excisional Biopsy:* removal of entire lump

What to Expect:

- Local anesthetic (you'll feel pressure, minimal pain)

- 15–30 minute procedure

- Possible bruising

The Phone Call

It was Friday, October 13th, 2006, just nine days after my 31st birthday. I had just pulled into a parking spot at Target, planning to run in quickly and grab a few things. Just a normal errand on an ordinary afternoon. Ever since my biopsy, I'd been trying to stay busy, keeping myself distracted with the little to-dos of everyday life so I wouldn't have to sit too long with the growing worry pressing into the corners of my mind.

Somewhere, in the black hole that was my purse, my cell phone began to ring. I fumbled through crumpled receipts, stray Goldfish crackers, loose change, and countless pens, trying to find the source of the ringing before it stopped. When I finally answered, I had no idea my entire life was about to change.

"Yes, hello?"

On the other end was my doctor, who wasted no time getting to the point. There was no gentle lead-in, no softening of the edges, no awkward small talk to brace me for what was coming. Her voice was steady, clinical, and utterly detached.

"Invasive ductal carcinoma. HER2-positive."

I blinked and felt a slow wave of static begin to creep across my brain. I had never heard of invasive ductal carcinoma, but I could tell by her tone of voice that it was serious. The words dropped around me like bricks, and I was suddenly weightless, drifting above myself while staring blankly at the steering wheel. I had no reference point for what she was saying. This was before smartphones, before Google lived in every pocket, and before you could search a medical term before you finished hearing it. I just sat there, heart pounding, while her words started to fade like they were far away, outside the car.

She just kept talking, rattling off more information that I couldn't process, and I only caught a few words here and there. The rest felt like smoke; thin, shapeless, impossible to hold onto. Finally, something inside me broke through the fog, and in a voice I barely recognized as my own, I cut in.

"Are you saying I have cancer?"

There was a pause, just long enough to confirm what I already knew in my gut. And then she said it plainly.

"Yes. I'm afraid I am."

She continued speaking, trying to explain what came next, but I couldn't hear a thing. My hands were shaking. My ears were ringing. The phone was still in my hand, but I felt like I was slipping through the cracks of reality. I don't know how long I sat there, just staring into space, but I knew something inside me had already shifted. That was the moment the version of me I'd always known, the carefree one, who believed that bad things happened to other people, began to fade. I wasn't gone, not yet, but I was already becoming someone else. I was caught in that strange in-between space, like a butterfly still tucked inside the chrysalis, unaware of how different everything would become.

Somehow, I managed to call my husband at work. And then I called my mom in Michigan. I couldn't tell you what I said. I'm sure my words were a tangled mess, falling out of my mouth before I could string them into proper sentences. It was pure word-vomit. If they asked questions, I doubt I gave answers. I didn't have any to give.

And then, as if my body couldn't quite comprehend the gravity of what had just happened, I did what I had planned to do all along. I went into Target.

I walked the aisles in a daze, picking up shampoo, fruit roll-ups, and paper towels. I moved through the motions like I always did, but nothing felt familiar. Everything looked the same, but the world had shifted under my feet. I don't remember the other shoppers. I don't remember the cashier. My body kept moving because my brain didn't know what else to do.

Not long after, my husband called me back. His voice was frantic, confused.

"Where are you? I rushed home and you're not here. I was worried."

"Oh," I replied, blinking like I'd just been shaken from a dream. "I'm at Target."

I genuinely didn't know what I was supposed to do next. Was he right? Should I have gone home? Maybe I should have curled up in a ball? Should I have started planning my next move? I had no idea what was appropriate in that moment. I didn't know how a newly diagnosed cancer patient was expected to act. So, I just... did what I already knew how to do.

That first week passed in a blur. A haze of appointments, unfamiliar terminology, and too many phone calls from numbers I didn't recognize. I didn't know how to schedule anything or what was urgent. I didn't understand how bad HER2-positive was, or what it meant. I didn't dare research it. I was too afraid to type the words into a search bar and see the worst-case scenarios staring back at me. So I waited. I sat by the phone, hoping someone would explain to me what to do, hoping someone would dig me out of the avalanche that had just buried my life.

The word *cancer* hits like a punch to the throat. The second you hear it, your brain starts to spiral. You imagine chemo. Baldness. Scars. Mastectomies. And yes, even death. Even if no one says it, you think about it. We all do, especially when we've never been through anything like this before.

What I wish someone had told me in those early moments is that **cancer isn't a one-size-fits-all diagnosis.** It's a scary word, but it doesn't always mean the worst-case scenario. There are so many different types of breast cancer, and just as many different treatment paths. Some cases require aggressive intervention, while others can be managed with surgery or hormone therapy alone. You might not need chemo. You might not need radiation. You might not need surgery. Every single person's journey is different from the next.

Your treatment will depend on your specific diagnosis—your type, grade, stage, genetic factors, medical history, and, believe it or not, *your choices*. You get a say in what happens next. And if your path doesn't look like someone else's, that doesn't make it wrong.

Take a moment to breathe. You don't have to understand it all today. You're not expected to have any answers, know what every medical term means or what comes next. All you need to know right now is that cancer is big. It's huge! But so is hope. And healing. And the power of finding the right people to walk alongside you.

Back in 2006, I had no idea how to find the people I needed. I was referred to a therapy group, but all I could envision was a group of old ladies, and I wasn't an old lady, so I never went. I didn't turn to the internet. I don't even know if Facebook groups existed at that time, but if they did, I certainly didn't join any. The only person I knew who had gone through breast cancer had been diagnosed twenty years earlier. She simply told me the chemo had made her very sick. I think she didn't want to scare me, and truthfully, I wasn't ready to hear much more.

Now, as I write this book, I've joined some of those Facebook groups to better understand what breast cancer patients are facing today. (My favorite is one called Breast Friends.) And while I've seen some amazing support systems and unbelievably kind people offering real help, I've also seen things that make my stomach turn. Some groups are flooded with spam, sketchy miracle cures, and people trying to make a profit off of fear and desperation. I've seen vulnerable women ask simple, honest questions and get swarmed with comments pushing supplements, teas, oils, and unproven treatments. It's infuriating.

My only advice is that if you're looking for support online, please be cautious. You deserve safe spaces and real answers. If a group feels overwhelming or leaves you more anxious than comforted, it's okay to walk away and try a different one. You do not owe anyone your time or your vulnerability. And if someone offers advice that could affect your treatment, even if it sounds amazing, please, always run it by your medical team first.

In a world of immediate answers and quick fixes, don't be fooled. I remember how raw I felt in those early days. How badly I wanted *something* to make it all feel less terrifying. And I completely understand the pull of a medicinal tea or a holistic diet, especially when you're drowning in the unknown. But there's a fine line between support and noise, and you don't need to sift through chaos to find clarity.

You deserve real connection and truth. And most of all, you deserve to be seen as a whole person, not just a diagnosis.

🧬 Understanding Your Diagnosis

Cancer Type	Key Characteristics
DCIS (In Situ)	Non-invasive, confined to ducts
IDC (Invasive Ductal Carcinoma)	Most common, spreads into nearby tissue
ILC (Invasive Lobular)	Starts in lobules; sometimes harder to detect
Triple-Negative	No ER/PR/HER2; aggressive, chemo-driven
HER2-Positive	Fast-growing; responds to targeted treatment
Hormone Receptor–Positive	Driven by estrogen/progesterone; treated with hormone blockers

💬 Quotes from Survivors

"I've always been a healthy, active person. I don't take any medications, I eat the best I can, and I walk at least two miles every day. I also get my routine mammogram every year."
—Sandra, diagnosed with breast cancer despite no symptoms

"I was a little nervous since I'd not had a mammogram before, but the technician who took care of me explained everything and made me feel comfortable. It was a great experience."
—Marilyn Alejandro-Rodriguez, diagnosed after her first mammogram

✒️ Chapter Highlights

- A routine exam can reveal serious concerns, even when no symptoms are present.

- Early imaging results may be inconclusive. Always follow up, even if reassured.

- A biopsy can be emotionally overwhelming, even when physically manageable.

- Patients can and should ask for anxiety support during procedures.

- "Cancer" is not a one-size-fits-all diagnosis; each case and treatment path is unique.

- Online communities can offer support, but it's important to approach them with caution.

🩶 Key Takeaway

This chapter holds space for the shock and fear that comes before the diagnosis. It's a reminder that it's okay to fall apart, to not know what to do, and to feel completely unprepared. You're not alone in that.

"I am proof that early detection works."
—*Olivia Newton-John;*
Promoted early detection, and founded a cancer and wellness research center in Melbourne, Australia.

3
Finding Your Voice in the Chaos

We sat there, my husband and I, in a cold, sterile exam room. The kind that hums with fluorescent light and smells faintly of antiseptic and anxiety. The air between us felt heavy, thick with tension and fear, as we waited for the surgeon to arrive. My husband had come with me to be my second set of ears, to help catch the details I might miss, and to ask the questions I hadn't yet thought to form. But when the doctor finally walked in, the entire energy in the room shifted, and not in the reassuring way we had hoped.

He didn't greet us. He didn't smile. He didn't even offer even the most basic courtesies that you'd expect from someone about to discuss major surgery and your future. Instead, he walked in briskly, opened my chart like he was reviewing my Amazon shopping list, and began speaking without so much as looking in our direction. There was no "How are you holding up?" No discussion of what to expect or how I was feeling. Just a clipped, impersonal announcement.

"We'll do a lumpectomy," he said, his voice flat and indifferent, as though he were reading off a menu.

That was it. One word. Dropped into the stillness like a stone into water, rippling outward in waves I wouldn't even begin to comprehend until later. There was no conversation about why that surgery was being recommended, no mention of alternatives, no explanation of the risks, and certainly nothing about what would happen afterward. No talk of reconstruction, healing, or even what recovery might entail. Just that one cold declaration, dropped like fact, as if my only role was to nod and comply without question.

I looked at my husband, and he looked back at me, both of us uncertain whether we were supposed to speak, or even what to say if we did. We had no idea what questions to ask because we hadn't been given enough information to know where to begin. We were brand new to this world of cancer and medicine, and we had naively hoped the

35

professionals would help guide us through it. But in that moment, we realized that, at least with this doctor, we were on our own.

The surgery was finally scheduled, a full month away. I felt the now-familiar pressure of panic rising up in my chest. I didn't know how aggressive the cancer was, or how quickly it could spread. I didn't know whether waiting that long was dangerous or if it would be okay. The doctor hadn't said, and to be honest, my survival seemed like a very low priority to him. My surgery felt more like an inconvenience interrupting his golf game, than an opportunity for him to save a life. My husband asked if there was any way to move it up sooner, and the response was a shrug from the staff at the front desk, as if we were asking for an earlier dinner reservation instead of a life-saving procedure. "That's the soonest we've got," they said. And that was the end of the conversation.

We left the hospital with a date on the calendar and a glossy brochure about lumpectomies in my hand. Outside, in the parking lot, I stood beside the car and let the tears fall, silently and without ceremony. I didn't have the words to describe what I was feeling. I just knew this was so big and I felt small, powerless, and unseen. I had gone into that office hoping for guidance, and a friendly face, but what I got was a stark reminder that, to some people, I was little more than a name on a chart. I wasn't a woman whose life had just been turned upside down. I was a file folder to be processed and moved along.

In that moment, I felt like my fear didn't matter to anyone. Like my voice didn't matter. Nobody but me gave a damn that I was drowning in a sea of medical jargon and institutional indifference, and I had no clue how to rescue myself. I know my family was effected, but they could walk away, go to work, go to school, and pretend this cancer didn't exist for a little while. I had no means of escape. I was completely alone.

What I didn't know then, but I do now, is that I wasn't alone. I had options. And so do you. It's important that you know and really understand that.

I didn't have to stay with that surgeon, and neither do you. I could have asked for a second opinion. I could have looked for a doctor who saw me as a person instead of a task. I could have demanded a conversation

36

instead of being handed a conclusion. I didn't realize that at the time, because I was scared and overwhelmed and trying to play by the rules of a system I didn't understand. But you don't have to make the same mistake I did. You can fight to be seen.

You deserve more than a shrug and a brochure. You deserve time, attention, explanation, and the ability to ask questions without feeling like a burden. If your doctor can't or won't provide that, then it is absolutely okay to find someone who will. This is your body. Your life. And your voice belongs in the room just as much as anyone else's.

Once you begin to find your footing, once you stop accepting indifference as the norm and start asking for what you need, the ground starts to gather back under your feet. The fear may not disappear, but the sense of powerlessness begins to lift. You may not be able to control everything about your diagnosis or your treatment, but you *can* control who you trust to walk beside you through it.

They say knowledge is power, and that's true, but so is the courage to speak up when something doesn't feel right. I want you to have all of it: the information, the confidence, and the clarity to move forward not as a passive patient, but as an active participant in your own care.

How to Speak Up for Yourself (Even When It's Hard)

Like a lot of little girls, I was taught to be quiet, polite, and agreeable. Respect your elders and all that jazz. I didn't want to question the experts, or be too difficult. But the thing I didn't realize is that cancer has nothing to do with being polite. Your life is at stake here and it's time to fight like hell. Create waves if you need to, to get answers and the help you deserve. The days of being polite are over.

You don't have to be loud to advocate for yourself, but you do have to be firm. State clearly that you have questions, concerns, and especially your boundaries. If you're like me, that's something that doesn't come naturally to you. Most of us aren't taught how to speak up in medical settings. We're taught to defer. After all, they're the professionals, right? But cancer changes the rules, and demands a seat at the table, and you deserve to sit in that seat fully informed and fully respected.

37

Here are a few ways to begin advocating for yourself, even if it feels uncomfortable:

- *Start by asking questions.* If your doctor explains something and you don't understand it, say so. For example, you might ask, "What are the pros and cons of lumpectomy versus mastectomy in my case?" or "If I delay surgery to think through my options, will it affect my outcome?" Questions like these can help you make choices that feel right for you, instead of being swept along by someone else's plan. Ask them to explain it in a different way. Say, "Can you walk me through what that means for me specifically?" or "Are there other options we haven't discussed yet?"

- *Bring someone with you.* Whether it's a friend, partner, or trusted family member, having someone else in the room can help you feel less alone, and they can speak up or take notes when your mind goes blank from stress.

- *Write things down.* Keep a notebook or use your phone to jot down questions before appointments if you need to. In the moment, it's easy to forget what you wanted to say. Having a list helps you stay focused and assertive.

- *Don't settle for being dismissed.* If a provider brushes off your concerns or talks down to you, that is not okay. Tell them, "I'm not comfortable with that," or "I'd like to get a second opinion." You do not need their permission to change doctors.

- *Practice saying things out loud.* It might sound silly, but rehearse phrases like "I'm not sure that's right for me" or "Can we talk about what this means long-term?" The more you practice, the more confident you'll feel.

- *Use your strength wisely.* Advocacy doesn't necessarily mean being aggressive or confrontational. But you do need to be firm. You can be kind and respectful and still demand the care you deserve. Those things are not mutually exclusive.

- *Do your research.* Learning about your diagnosis, surgery options, and possible side effects can help you feel more in control. Ask your care team if they have a printable checklist of questions to bring to consultations, or if there's a patient navigator available—someone who can walk with you through the decision-making process and explain things clearly. Don't be afraid to bring up what you've read or ask for clarification if things don't make sense. Sites like Breastcancer.org and the American Cancer Society are great places to start, and your hospital's patient education department may also have helpful booklets or videos.

- *Don't be afraid to get a second opinion.* A different doctor may offer a different perspective, more options, or a better bedside manner. If something doesn't sit right with you, trust that feeling. You deserve care that makes you feel seen, heard, and safe.

One woman I talked to said, "I've had to yell louder than my doctors just to be heard." And that is just bananas to me. You shouldn't have to fight to be seen. But if you do find yourself in that position, please know that speaking up is not selfish. We all must do what needs to be done for our survival.

As the patient, you are the most important person in that room. Remember that! You're not asking for too much. You're asking for your life, and that's always worth raising your voice for. If your doctor doesn't respect that, then find another doctor.

Understanding Your Surgical Options

When people hear "breast cancer surgery," the first thing they think of is a mastectomy. But the reality is more nuanced, and your surgical path might look very different from someone else's.

There are two main types of breast cancer surgery: **lumpectomy** and **mastectomy**. Both can be incredibly effective, but what's "best" depends on your diagnosis, your care team's recommendations, and your personal values and preferences.

⚕ Lumpectomy: Breast-Conserving Surgery

A lumpectomy removes the cancer and a small rim of healthy tissue around it, often leaving the majority of the breast intact. Recovery is usually shorter, and many people go home the same day. You may feel physically functional within a week or two, but it's still major surgery. Your body is being changed, and it's okay to grieve that.

Even though the physical change may seem small, the emotional impact can still be profound. You may look at your body and feel different, unsure, or even a little disconnected. These reactions are normal.

⚕ Mastectomy: Total Breast Removal

A mastectomy involves removing all of the breast tissue from one or both breasts. There are variations—skin-sparing, nipple-sparing, bilateral—but in all cases, it's a much more intense surgery physically and emotionally.

Some people feel empowered by the choice to "take it all." Others experience grief, sadness, or a deep sense of loss. And many feel a mixture of both. Whether you choose mastectomy out of necessity or preference, your feelings are valid.

It's important to remember that even when a surgeon tells you what they recommend, you still have a right to ask, "What are my other options?" For example: "If a mastectomy is being recommended, is there a reason lumpectomy wouldn't be appropriate in my case? What are the risks and benefits of each?"

If you're not getting clear answers, or the conversation feels rushed or dismissive, that's your cue to pause and advocate for yourself. You deserve to feel confident in your care plan, and you're allowed to ask for more information, or even a second opinion, before making a choice that will impact the rest of your life.

✎ Belinda C., Diagnosed at 67

Belinda had no symptoms—no lump, no pain. Just a routine mammogram. The results came back questionable, so they sent her for more tests. Then a biopsy. And then came the waiting. She was in that awful space between what you hope is nothing and what your gut quietly suspects, filled with the low, steady hum of "what if."

When her doctor finally called, she told Belinda over the phone: invasive ductal carcinoma, triple positive. The tumor was small, only half a centimeter, and caught early. That should have brought some comfort, but hearing those words still knocked the wind right out of her. Belinda sat there for a long time, numb, and then the tears came, quiet and unstoppable. She didn't pick up the phone to call anyone. She just couldn't. All she could do was text her adult children, and her grandson, because she was still just trying to remember how to breathe. She needed space to process what she had just learned.

From that moment forward, life became a blur of appointments— bloodwork, consultations, questions she didn't yet know how to ask. Belinda met with the oncologist, then the surgeon. The initial plan felt manageable: a lumpectomy followed by radiation. The surgery was scheduled for June 3rd, and she started to believe that maybe she could walk through this without too much disruption. But when she returned for the follow-up appointment, everything changed.

The pathology report showed something new—DCIS—and one of the margins wasn't clear. Even the surgeon and pathologist were surprised. Just like that, her plan unraveled. Belinda was told she'd need another surgery, and now, chemotherapy too.

That word, *chemo*, hit her like a brick to the chest. She said she cried the entire day. She wasn't prepared for how quickly things shifted, how easily every bit of good news could be erased in a single sentence. Her gut had been whispering all along: *Get the mastectomy.* She said she had been brushing it aside, but this time, she said it out loud. She told the nurse navigator, and thankfully, she didn't dismiss Belinda. She listened and heard Belinda's feelings. The nurse navigator honored Belinda's instinct. She was scheduled to have her right breast removed in July. It wasn't the original plan, but it's the decision that helps Belinda sleep at night.

41

For her, the hardest part isn't the logistics. She talks about the fear. How it's always there, even when it's quiet. How it settles into your bones, sits behind your eyes, clings to your thoughts when you're trying to fall asleep. She told me how she's scared of chemo. Scared of what's still ahead. People don't understand that the fear doesn't go away after the diagnosis. It just changes shape. You don't stop being afraid. You just learn how to function around it.

These days, she tries to take it one step at a time. She spends her time listening to comedy podcasts on the drive to appointments, trying to shake loose the tension that builds up in her chest. She lets herself cry when she needs to. She tries to stay present, to feel whatever the moment is offering, because even now, even in the middle of the fear, she wants to just feel alive.

🌀 Discussing Reconstruction

Some women choose to have reconstruction right away, while others wait, and some opt not to have it at all. Every decision is valid, and there is no single "right" path—only what feels right for you.

Reconstruction can involve:

- **Implants** (saline or silicone)

- **Autologous tissue** (using fat and muscle from another part of your body, like a DIEP flap or TRAM flap)

- **A combination of both**

🧩 Implant-Based Reconstruction

This is often done in stages. First, tissue expanders are inserted to gradually stretch the chest wall. Once the skin is ready, they're replaced with permanent implants. This method can be less invasive upfront, with a shorter initial recovery time. But implants aren't always a one-and-done solution—many women eventually need revisions or replacements.

Some people experience tightness, rippling, or changes in sensation. Implants can also impact posture and sleep, and in rare cases, can lead to complications like capsular contracture, where scar tissue hardens around the implant.

Autologous Tissue Reconstruction

Also known as flap reconstruction, this technique uses your own body tissue (often from your belly, thigh, or back) to form a new breast mound. Common types include:

- **DIEP flap**: Uses abdominal skin and fat, sparing the muscle.

- **TRAM flap**: Uses abdominal muscle along with skin and fat.

- **Latissimus dorsi flap**: Uses muscle and tissue from your back.

These surgeries take longer, with more involved recovery, and can come with complications in both the breast and donor site. But many women feel the results look and feel more natural—sometimes even warm to the touch, unlike implants.

How Radiation Affects Reconstruction

Radiation can change the texture and elasticity of your skin. It can delay healing and increase the risk of infection. It also makes implants more likely to harden or shift. That's why many doctors recommend delaying implant reconstruction until after radiation, or choosing flap reconstruction, which tends to tolerate radiation better.

If radiation is part of your treatment plan, be sure to ask your doctor about how it will affect reconstruction options. Sometimes it's best to place a temporary spacer, or wait entirely.

Going Flat Is an Option, Too

For some women, the thought of more surgery, more recovery, and more trauma to an already exhausted body just doesn't feel worth it—and so they choose to skip reconstruction entirely and go flat. This is not because they're giving up. In fact, for many, it's the exact opposite. Choosing to go flat is about taking back control in a situation that feels completely out of their hands. It's about saying, "I've been through enough, and I get to decide what happens next."

Some women go flat from day one, knowing that it's the best decision for their body and their peace of mind. Others start with one plan and change course somewhere along the way. Some wear prosthetics when they want to. Others don't bother. Some adorn their scars with tattoos, turning their bodies into living, breathing works of art; symbols of survival and reclamation.

The point is this: **you have choices.**

And you deserve the truth about those choices, not just a glossy pamphlet shoved into your hands, or a two-minute conversation that skips over anything that doesn't involve implants. You have every right to ask your surgeon to slow down and explain *everything*. Every option. Every risk. Every possible outcome. Ask for photos. Ask for patient stories. Ask about recovery times, possible complications, and what life might look like five or ten years down the road. If they aren't willing to take the time to answer your questions, then it might be time to consider a different surgeon.

This is your body and your healing. This is your life moving forward. You are the one who gets to choose the path that feels right, whether it's flat, reconstructed, tattooed, scarred, or completely undecided for now.

Whatever you decide, make that decision with your eyes open, your voice heard, and your heart centered in what matters most. Because there's no one-size-fits-all version of healing. There's just you, and the strength you bring to every single step.

💔 The Emotional Impact of Surgery

These surgeries can hugely affect your identity and sense of self. For many women, the breasts are such an integral part of their womanhood. The changes to your body are real, and when you undergo such invasive surgeries, the effects are so much deeper than physical scars.

Your breasts may be part of your femininity, your intimacy, your motherhood, your confidence. Losing them, or even changing them, can feel like losing a large part of yourself, and the grief that follows is real and normal.

You might feel:

- Grief over how you used to look or feel

- Anger that you didn't get to choose this path

- Discomfort or awkwardness during intimacy

- Disconnected from your body, like it no longer feels like "yours"

These are all normal, natural feelings. Please know that you're not alone in any of this.

Talk to a therapist if you need help. Ask your doctor for a referral. Reach out to other survivors who've walked this road. Give yourself time. These changes are so emotional, and you deserve reassurance and support to get through to the other side.

✎ Andrea H., Diagnosed at 59

When Andrea was first diagnosed, they told her that she had three masses in her right breast. The surgeon was confident he could remove them all with a lumpectomy. They were close together, and the plan seemed straightforward. But when the MRI came back, there was a fourth mass in the right breast, and three more in the left. That changed everything.

Andrea didn't want to wait around for more biopsies. She was already feeling overwhelmed, and exhausted. She told her surgeon that she wanted a double mastectomy. Just take it all. She needed to feel like she was making the call, not just reacting to bad news on repeat.

So, they scheduled the surgery and Andrea decided on immediate reconstruction. That part gave her hope. She thought, maybe she would still look like herself. But weeks later, the left side failed and the implant had to be removed. She told herself they would fix it. But then the right side failed, too. Another surgery. More healing. More loss.

Andrea said she never expected to be flat. She never imagined waking up and seeing a body in the mirror that didn't feel like her own anymore.

That was one of the darkest parts of the journey for her. Not just physically, but emotionally. She said she felt erased. She didn't recognize herself. Didn't feel feminine. Or strong. There was no warning for how hard that grief would hit her, and no one around really knew what to say.

Andrea tells me that she felt like she was losing herself in pieces, first the diagnosis, then her breasts, then her plans. Some days she said she wanted to fight. Other days she didn't want to get out of bed at all. The emotional whiplash made her feel like everything was coming undone. But she knew she couldn't stay there.

Fortunately, she reached out for help; therapy, meditation, support groups. Her husband was steady and kind through all of it. She prayed. And gave herself permission to not be okay. That was new for her. She says, "I stopped pretending I was fine and started giving myself grace instead."

Andrea says that cancer has changed her. She doesn't rush anymore. She listens to her body, and spirit. She does what feels right and lets that be enough.

✎ Ellen C., Diagnosed at 57

Ellen was 57 when she was diagnosed with DCIS, stage 0, but with a high grade. At the time, she was dealing with heart issues and had put off mammograms for years. When she finally went in, she wasn't expecting much. But that first scan led to another, and then a biopsy. On January 13th, they called with the bombshell.

Ellen says, "I remember feeling completely numb. Detached. Like I was watching someone else go through it all from outside of my body. More biopsies followed, and the final decision came down to a double mastectomy. I didn't want radiation or hormone blockers if I could help it. It just felt like too much for my body to handle on top of everything else. The surgery confirmed it was the right call. There was a small invasive tumor, and my 'healthy' breast wasn't so healthy after all."

46

Physically, Ellen says that the recovery was easier than she expected. But she felt off-balance, literally and figuratively. She'd spent her life with very large breasts. Suddenly, they were gone. And she said she didn't know how to feel like a woman anymore.

Breasts carry so much of our identity. Our femininity. The absence of them can feel like an absence of *you*. That was the hardest part, grieving something the world tells you not to grieve.

Ellen says she's still in expanders now, and jokes that she's on the "Free the Foobs Summer Tour '25." She says her $80 bras have been replaced with joy over $10 ones, or none at all.

But behind the humor is real change. Spiritually, she has found herself praying more. And emotionally, she's had to admit something that's always been hard: she needed help.

"That's one of the things cancer teaches you," Ellen says. "You don't get to do it all alone. Some of the people I expected to show up didn't. And some I never saw coming were right there when I needed them. My husband, my son, my friends, even my rescue dog, all of them carried me when I couldn't carry myself. And God. He's been with me through every single step of the way."

"I still get scared," Ellen continues. "Every ache, every new sensation, brings a whisper of fear. But I'm more mindful now. I treat myself with kindness. I cry when I need to. And I laugh. A lot."

If Ellen could share any advice, it would be this:
"Give yourself grace. This isn't a sprint, it's a marathon.
Don't compare your healing to anyone else's. Let it be yours alone.
And join the support groups. Your pink sisters *will* help you through."

Questions to Ask Your Surgeon

About Options & Decisions:

- What are my surgical options, and why are you recommending one over the others?

- Can I safely delay surgery to seek a second opinion or process my options?

- Will I need additional treatments afterward (like radiation or chemotherapy)?

- What happens if I choose not to reconstruct at all?

- How might radiation affect my surgical outcome or future reconstruction?

About Recovery & Life After:

- What is the expected recovery time for each option?

- Will I have drains, and how long will they need to stay in?

- Will I regain sensation in my chest? If not, what should I expect that to feel like?

- How will this affect future imaging, monitoring, or screenings?

- Are there physical limitations I should expect (lifting, sleeping positions, exercise)?

- What kind of scarring should I expect — both from the breast area and possible donor sites?

About Reconstruction:

- What reconstruction options are available — immediate, delayed, or none?

- Can I meet with a plastic surgeon before making my decision?

- What are the possible complications or revision rates for each reconstruction type?

- How does radiation influence the success or risks of implant vs. flap reconstruction?

- Will implants need to be replaced later in life?

About Their Experience:

- How many of these specific procedures have you performed?

- What outcomes have your patients experienced (both physical and emotional)?

- Can you provide any written materials, photos, or diagrams to review at home?

Insurance & Support:

- Will insurance cover surgery and reconstruction?

- Are there costs I should be prepared for outside of what insurance covers?

- Is emotional or psychological support available before or after surgery?

- Can I be connected with a counselor, support group, or patient navigator?

Waiting for Surgery: A Storm of Emotions

For me, that stretch of time between diagnosis and surgery was easily one of the hardest parts of the whole damn thing.

I felt like I was dangling in limbo, with nothing solid to hold onto. No answers. No control. Just an endless countdown to a surgery date that felt too far away. And during that time, my husband—bless him—was doing everything he knew how to do. He was a doer. A fixer. The kind of guy who doesn't sit still well, especially when someone he loves is hurting. So every day, like clockwork, he called the hospital. He asked for updates. Pushed for earlier appointments. Demanded answers from schedulers who probably hated seeing his name on caller ID.

He was trying to fight against the system, trying to bulldoze through the uncertainty, because he didn't know how to fight the fear.

And I knew that. I really did. I saw that it was his panic dressed up in action. It was the only way he knew how to cope. He needed to help.

But the more he did, the more my anxiety went up. His urgency didn't calm me, it ramped everything up. It kept all my worries in the forefront of my mind. Every time he paced or made another phone call or ranted about the hospital's scheduling system, it felt like the thin ground beneath us cracked a little wider. I could feel both of us falling into that dark pit of helplessness, and it was exhausting.

What I really needed most from him in those moments wasn't action. I didn't need someone to fix it, or fight the calendar, or demand a plan that hadn't been formed yet. I just needed him to sit next to me, take my hand, and say, "This sucks, but I'm here. We'll face it together." That's it. Not a heroic rescue. Just presence. Steadiness. A place to land.

But I didn't know how to ask for that. I didn't want to hurt his feelings or make him feel unappreciated, so I said nothing. I let him run full-speed into logistics and phone calls and hospital red tape while I silently crumbled on the inside. I knew he was doing it out of love and concern. I knew his heart was in the right place. And I didn't want to dim the only thing that gave him a sense of control.

Years later, I've looked back at that version of him, panicked, helpless, trying like hell to be useful, and I see just how scared he must have been. Maybe even more scared than I was. Because at least I had something to fight. I had doctor's appointments and scans and surgery on the horizon. I had a path, even if it was terrifying. But he had nothing to hold onto. No battle plan. No checklist. No clear way to protect me. Just fear and silence and the unbearable weight of watching someone he loves walk into a storm he couldn't stop.

And I get it now. That helplessness is its own kind of pain. It doesn't get talked about enough, but it's real, and it deserves some grace.

Coping While You Wait

That stretch of time between diagnosis and surgery can feel like a no-man's-land. You've received life-changing news, but the action hasn't started yet. It's a strange place to be—uncertain, powerless, and often overlooked.

The quiet waiting is where anxiety can take hold. Your mind might spiral with what-ifs, and your body may carry tension in ways you don't even recognize. Here are some tips to help you manage this emotional holding pattern:

Choose the Right Advocate
Your partner might not always be the best choice. That's okay. Choose someone who brings calm, clarity, and confidence to your appointments. You need someone who can listen, take notes, and ask thoughtful questions without adding to your stress.

Write Your Questions Down
Between your appointments, keep a running list of questions in your phone or a notebook. Don't try to remember everything in the moment —stress has a way of making your brain go blank. This list will help you feel grounded and prepared.

Ask for a Patient Navigator
Many hospitals have a breast cancer patient navigator—a nurse or social worker who specializes in helping patients understand their diagnosis and treatment path. Ask if this is available to you. They can explain things in plain language, help coordinate appointments, and advocate on your behalf.

Make Use of Printables and Tools
Ask your hospital if they offer a printable question checklist, or bring one of your own. Having something tangible in your hand can help keep the conversation focused and ensure you don't leave without the answers you need.

Seek Counseling, Together or Alone
Therapy isn't just for after treatment, and it isn't only for the patient. It can be incredibly helpful right now. If you're in a relationship, consider couples counseling. Many couples find themselves struggling to communicate during this time, either trying to protect each other from fear or simply speaking different emotional languages. Therapy gives you tools to meet each other where you are.

Handle Practical Matters Sooner Than Later
This might be a good time to address legal documents like a will, medical power of attorney, or advance directives. Having these conversations now might bring peace of mind later, knowing that

you've taken steps to protect yourself and your loved ones. It also helps keep your mind on other things while you wait.

Let Yourself Nest
You might find yourself suddenly cleaning out closets, organizing drawers, or obsessively meal-prepping. That's okay. Your brain is trying to create control and order where it can. Lean into it. This is one way your body is protecting you.

Make Room for Joy
Watch a funny show, bake something you love, get outside in the sun, or start a creative project. These aren't just distractions, they're healing acts. Laughter, creativity, and connection help your nervous system find peace, even in the middle of waiting.

Give Yourself Permission to Feel
You don't need to be brave all the time. It's okay to be scared, angry, overwhelmed, or numb. You're allowed to have your own reaction, in your own time. Cry if you need to. Talk if you're ready. Retreat if it helps. There's no wrong way to feel.

Final Stories & Reflections

Tina B., Diagnosed at 62
"The hardest part wasn't the surgery. It was waking up afterward and feeling like I didn't know the body I was living in anymore. I had always been curvy. Always worn bold colors and low-cut blouses. I felt invisible for a long time after. But slowly, I started seeing the strength in my reflection. I dressed in ways that made me feel like me again. I wore scarves and earrings and bold lipstick. I built a new relationship with my body, not based on how it looked, but how it carried me through something unimaginable."

Rebecca J., Diagnosed at 35
"Being diagnosed so young was a shock. I had just gotten married, we were talking about kids. My mind went into a spiral of all the things I might not get to do. I chose a double mastectomy with no reconstruction. It was the right choice for me, but explaining that to people was exhausting. I got so many comments like, 'But you're so young,' or 'You'll change your mind.' But I didn't. I found power in the

decision to live without breasts. It doesn't make me less of a woman. If anything, I feel more grounded in who I am now."

Melinda K., Diagnosed at 47

"I struggled for a long time after my lumpectomy. Everyone acted like it wasn't a big deal because I 'got to keep my breast.' But it didn't feel like mine anymore. There was a chunk missing, and a scar, and my clothes fit weird, and I felt broken. It wasn't until I joined a support group that I heard someone else say the same thing. That's when I realized how much I needed to hear it wasn't just me. The surgery saved my life, yes. But it also changed it. Both things can be true."

Lynn G., Diagnosed at 58

"If I could say anything to someone just starting this journey, it would be this: Bring someone with you to every appointment. Ask questions. Take notes. Push for answers. You'll need advocates. You'll need strength you didn't know you had. And be prepared. The support at the beginning can fade. But you have to keep showing up. Even when you're scared. Even when you're tired."

"You don't owe the world a brave face every day," Lynn continues. "Let yourself feel it all. Let yourself be honest. Because this road is long, and the fear, especially the fear of what might still be lurking, doesn't just disappear. But neither does your strength."

Chapter Highlights

- You have options. If your doctor doesn't explain them or treat you with respect, you are allowed to switch providers.

- There are two main surgical paths: lumpectomy and mastectomy. Both are valid, and neither is one-size-fits-all.

- Reconstruction is optional, and comes with physical, emotional, and long-term considerations.

- Radiation can affect healing and reconstruction outcomes, especially with implants.

- Advocacy is not about being aggressive. It's about being clear, informed, and standing up for your own care.

- The emotional impact of breast surgery is profound and valid. Grief, anger, and body disconnect are common and deserve support.

🤍 **Key Takeaway**

This chapter is about reclaiming your voice in a system that can make you feel invisible. You are not just a diagnosis. You are a whole person, and your choices deserve to be honored with care, compassion, and clarity.

"Cancer didn't take me down. It taught me to look at life differently."
—Suzanne Somers; Advocated for alternative/integrative treatment approaches

4
The Cut That Heals

I woke up in the recovery room with a throat that felt like sandpaper and vision that blurred at the edges. For a moment, I wasn't sure where I was or why everything felt so heavy. But then it came back to me. The surgery was over. The tumor had been removed. I had done it. I had taken the first step towards taking back control of my life.

I actually thought the hardest part was behind me. I believed, naively, that cutting out the cancer was the victory lap. The danger was out and I could finally breathe again.

No one had warned me how wrong I was. No one had explained to me about what comes after.

Once I got home, everything seemed to go quiet. For the first time in weeks, the whirlwind of tests, scans, and scheduling finally slowed down. My body was sore, but there was this strange sense of peace. I really believed I was past the worst of it. That we'd pulled the poison out of my body and now I could rest, heal, and move forward.

Then the call came.

It had been about a week since the surgery, and the moment I saw the caller ID, I felt sick to my stomach. The lab results were back, and just like that, the ground shifted out from under me again. The margins around the tumor weren't clear. They hadn't gotten it all. I'd need another surgery.

Panic hit me like a freight train. I had barely begun to process the first procedure, and now we were doing it all over again. It felt like being shoved back to square one. Worse, actually, because now I knew what recovery felt like, and I wasn't exactly eager to do it again.

And that wasn't all. During the first surgery, they had removed a few lymph nodes from under my arm to check for spread. Two out of three came back positive. I didn't fully understand what that meant at the time, because once the doctor started talking about nodes, margins, staging, and grades, it all blurred into static. I hadn't gone to medical school. I wasn't equipped to speak fluent oncology.

All I could process was this: cancer in my lymph nodes. And that scared the absolute hell out of me.

Looking back now, I feel like only two positive nodes was actually good news. It meant we had caught it just in time. But when you're sitting there, still stitched together and emotionally unraveling, all you hear is *more cancer*. You don't hear "caught early." You don't hear "manageable." You only hear "still there."

If you're in that place right now, confused, numb, terrified, I want you to hear me clearly: *You're not alone*. I've been there too. Most of us have. You're not stupid for not understanding all the medical terms. You're not weak for crying when you hear words you don't fully grasp. You probably didn't go to medical school, so why would you know those terms? Take it slow. You're doing the best you can in a completely overwhelming situation.

🔍 What to Expect After Surgery

The days after surgery are often filled with a quiet that feels unfamiliar. You're not rushing to appointments or tests. You're waiting. Watching. Healing. But even this part carries uncertainty, because healing isn't always linear. You might be sore, groggy, and confused. You might be grieving what was taken from your body. Or you might feel nothing at all.

🏥 Common Procedures Recap

- **Lumpectomy** removes only the tumor and a margin of surrounding tissue.

- **Mastectomy** removes one or both breasts, sometimes including chest muscle depending on severity.

- **Sentinel node biopsy** checks the first few lymph nodes for signs of spread.

- **Axillary node dissection** removes more nodes if cancer is found in the sentinel group.

- **Re-excision** is a second surgery to remove more tissue if margins weren't clear.

Key Terms

- **Margins:** The edge of the tissue removed during surgery. "Clear" margins mean no cancer cells are found at the outer edge. If they're not clear, another surgery may be needed.

- **Lymphedema:** Swelling that can happen when lymph nodes are removed or damaged, affecting fluid drainage.

- **Re-excision:** A follow-up surgery to remove more tissue when initial margins were not clear.

Questions to Ask Before Leaving the Hospital

- How many lymph nodes were removed, and were any positive?

- Were my margins clear?

- Will I need a re-excision?

- What pain medications are prescribed, and what should I expect?

- How should I care for my incision and any drains?

- Are there signs of infection I should watch for?

- What activities should I avoid in the next few weeks?

- When is my follow-up appointment?

- Who should I contact with urgent questions, during business hours and after hours?

Quotes from Survivors

"The biggest thing I had to learn after surviving breast cancer was how I felt about 'beauty.' Feeling beautiful didn't mean having the perfect body or the perfect hair. Beauty isn't perfection. Strength is." —Alex, post-mastectomy

"I feel more confident in myself for what I've been through. Breast cancer doesn't have to take away your beauty and femininity." — Margee, bilateral mastectomy with reconstruction

"I realized in November after a haircut that I liked it! Beauty to me is learning to embrace my scars and what I look like today, not what I looked like before cancer or what I want to look like. Just simply embracing today." —Angie, embracing her post-surgery body

Common Post-Surgical Experiences & Tips

From stiffness and swelling to emotional whiplash, recovery often comes with more questions than answers. Some women feel stronger right away. Others experience numbness, phantom pain, or emotional grief over what's been lost.

Pam shared

"I had a lumpectomy with clear margins, but my whole chest felt different," Pam shares. "I couldn't explain it. It wasn't just the physical healing. It was the mental fog that came with it. I felt like I had no right to be sad because I 'only' had a lumpectomy."

Breast cancer isn't about comparison. Grief isn't a contest. Whether your surgery was "minor" or extensive, you are still allowed to feel it all. There is no hierarchy in pain, and no shame in needing time to process what just happened to your body.

Victoria G., Diagnosed at 67

Victoria was 67 when she found a lump. That was in early November. The radiologist called her back for a follow-up, and on November 25th, they confirmed what she'd been dreading. It was cancer. Left breast. Her surgeon offered a choice of a lumpectomy or a single mastectomy. Victoria told her surgeon, without hesitation: take them both.

The surgeon asked if Victoria wanted reconstruction, and she said, "This will probably shock you, but my modeling days are over. Just take them and leave me flat." No hesitation, and no back and forth. She just wanted them gone.

That same week, her family sent her on a cruise. They timed it so she would be getting back just three days before her double mastectomy. So there she was, sitting on a beach looking out at the beautiful ocean, and something came over her. "I thought, *You know what, Victoria? Quit feeling sorry for yourself.* It's not your arms or your legs. You're not losing your eyesight. You don't have ALS. Knock it off."

So, Victoria says, "that cruise became my 'ta-ta to the ta-tas.'"

Looking back, Victoria's favorite piece of advice is this: **trust your gut.** Her first oncologist was stiff, clinical, and got *visibly annoyed* with her when she cried during an appointment. She walked out and never went back.

Her second oncologist listened. She cared.

Victoria reminds us, "Don't let anyone make you feel like you have to fit a mold. For me, losing my breasts wasn't the end of anything. It was a new beginning. I kept my humor, held on to my dignity, and gained a whole lot of strength along the way."

◊ Understanding Lymphedema

Doctors often begin by checking whether breast cancer has reached the lymphatic system. The lymph nodes—particularly those under the arm—act like small security checkpoints. If cancer is found there, it can be an early indicator that the disease may be starting to spread.

Dana shared, "I didn't even know what lymph nodes really did until mine were gone. I had five removed, and now my left arm gets puffy after walking the dog. I wear a compression sleeve and it helps. But it was a complete surprise. I wish I'd known what to watch for.

Understanding the lymphatic system, and how it might respond after surgery, helps you spot issues before they grow into long-term complications.

🌢 Why Lymph Nodes Are Tested — and How Their Removal Can Affect You

When breast cancer is diagnosed, one of the most important things your medical team needs to know is whether the cancer has spread beyond the breast itself. The **lymphatic system** is one of the first places cancer cells may travel, and the lymph nodes under your arm, called the **axillary lymph nodes**, are the most common first stop. These tiny, bean-shaped glands act like security checkpoints. Their job is to filter out harmful substances, including cancer cells, so testing them can reveal a lot about how far your cancer may have progressed.

The first step in checking for spread is usually a **sentinel lymph node biopsy**. During this surgery, a tracer dye is injected near the tumor site. This dye helps the surgeon locate the "sentinel" nodes, which are the first few lymph nodes that drain fluid from the breast. These are removed and then closely examined under a microscope. If no cancer is found in those sentinel nodes, it's a good sign the cancer hasn't moved beyond the breast.

However, if cancer cells are found in those initial nodes, the next step may be an **axillary lymph node dissection**. This is a more extensive surgery where several more lymph nodes are removed to better understand how far the disease has spread. While this surgery gives doctors critical insight into your treatment needs, it also comes with long-term risks.

🌢 Understanding Secondary Lymphedema

One of the most common complications after lymph node removal or radiation is a condition called **secondary lymphedema**. Unlike primary lymphedema, which is a rare inherited condition, *secondary* lymphedema develops as a direct result of damage to the lymphatic system, which is something that happens frequently during cancer treatment.

When your lymph nodes are removed or damaged, the normal flow of lymphatic fluid can become disrupted. Instead of draining smoothly through your system, that fluid can get backed up, usually in the arm, hand, breast, or chest wall on the side of surgery. This build-up causes **chronic swelling** that can range from mild puffiness to significant, painful enlargement.

What makes this especially frustrating is that **secondary lymphedema can show up weeks, months, or even years after treatment ends**. And once it develops, there's no permanent cure. All you can do is try to manage it. That's why **early awareness and prevention are key**.

▶ Signs to Watch For

One of the hardest things about lymphedema is that it doesn't always happen right away. It can creep in slowly, weeks or even years after surgery or radiation. That's why it's so important to know what to watch for. Your body will often whisper before it shouts.

You might notice a strange heaviness or tightness in your arm, chest, or hand. It's subtle at first, like your sleeve fits just a little more snugly than it used to, or your ring doesn't slide on quite the same way. Maybe your skin feels a little firmer or warmer to the touch, or your range of motion isn't what it once was. Some people describe a tingling sensation, like their arm is falling asleep. These early signs may come and go at first, but they're worth paying attention to. Again, you know your body. Trust your instincts.

If you notice any of these things, don't brush it off. Speak up and ask your doctor for a referral to a certified lymphedema therapist. That is someone who specializes in managing and treating these exact symptoms. The sooner you get help, the more manageable it tends to be.

🛡 Prevention and Daily Care

If you've had lymph nodes removed or received radiation near your lymphatic system, there are some small ways you can protect yourself from developing lymphedema, or at least help keep it from getting worse if it does happen.

61

Try to avoid any medical procedures like blood pressure checks, IVs, or blood draws on the side of your body where the nodes were removed. It might seem like a little thing, but those small choices can reduce your risk of irritation or infection. Keep your skin healthy and moisturized, especially in that area. Even a tiny cut or nick while shaving can open the door for infection, so use caution. And if you're doing chores like gardening or cleaning, consider wearing gloves to protect your hands and arms from scratches or exposure to harsh chemicals.

Heat can be a trigger for some people, so hot tubs, saunas, or even very hot baths may increase the chance of swelling. So if you notice that you're more swollen after those activities, listen to the signal that your body is giving and adjust as needed. And while staying active is encouraged, try to ease into exercise gently. Repetitive motion or heavy lifting too soon can strain your lymphatic system.

Some survivors find that wearing a compression sleeve helps, especially during long flights or days when they're on their feet more than usual. That's something to talk through with your care team or a lymphedema specialist, because what works best is different for everyone.

Finally, and most importantly, if you ever notice redness, warmth, or a sudden spike in swelling, especially if it comes with a fever, that could be a sign of infection. Call your doctor immediately, don't wait. The faster you react to these things, the easier they are to take care of.

You deserve to feel safe and cared for in your body. Knowing how to protect your lymphatic system so important and shouldn't be overlooked. It's one more way to walk forward in healing, informed and supported.

You Are Not Alone

Lymphedema can feel like a cruel reminder of what you've survived, but please know that there is help. There are so many people who understand this condition and are trained to help you live a full life, with or without swelling. You can ask questions, ask for support, and even grieve the changes in your life. You're still every bit as strong, beautiful, and capable as you were before. Now that you know the signs and the steps, you're better equipped to take care of yourself.

▐▌ Understanding Tumor Grade & Stage

After my tumor was removed and sent to pathology, my doctor was finally able to give me some answers. He talked about things like the *grade* and *stage* of my tumor. Of course I had no idea what any of it meant, but once he broke it down, I started to understand how they helped with shaping what came next in my treatment plan.

Let's start with **tumor grade**. This is all about what the cancer cells look like under a microscope. Pathologists are basically looking at how "normal" or "abnormal" the cells appear and trying to predict how quickly they might grow or spread. If the cells look pretty close to normal breast cells and aren't dividing very fast, that's a low-grade tumor; referred to as Grade 1. These usually grow slowly. Grade 2 means the cells look a bit more off, and they're growing at a moderate pace. Grade 3 is when the cells look very different and are more likely to be aggressive. Mine fell somewhere in the middle, which felt both reassuring and unsettling.

If you're in this boat, ask your doctor, "What grade is my tumor, and how does that affect my treatment?" It's a simple question, but the answer gives a lot of insight into how serious things are and what kind of response your team is planning.

Then there's the **stage**, which is a different kind of measurement. While grade is about the behavior of the cells, *stage* is about how far the cancer has already traveled. It looks at both the size of the tumor and whether or not it's moved into lymph nodes, or even other parts of the body.

Stage 0 means the cancer hasn't spread beyond where it started. It's very early and non-invasive. Stage I is still early but might involve a small lump that's localized. Stage II might mean the tumor is larger or it's reached a few nearby lymph nodes. Stage III is more advanced, maybe affecting more nodes or nearby tissue, but it's still considered regional. Stage IV means the cancer has traveled to distant parts of the body like the bones or lungs.

Again, a good question to ask is, "What stage is my cancer, and what does that mean for treatment and follow-up?" These two things, grade and stage, don't tell the whole story, but they help your care team figure out the best way to move forward.

But here's something really important, and I need to say this clearly: **cancer is cancer**, no matter the grade or stage. One woman I spoke with said, "I wish people understood that even if it's Stage 0, it's *still* cancer. The fear, the anxiety, and the stress are all still there. Don't dismiss someone else's experience just because it's not 'advanced.'" And she was absolutely right. Every diagnosis hits hard. Every single person deserves support, compassion, and room to process what they're going through. Your feelings are valid, no matter the report, or what that annoying coworker, says.

✅ Chapter Highlights

- Clear surgical margins mean no cancer cells at the tissue's edge. If they're not clear, a second surgery (re-excision) may be needed.

- Lymph node removal helps determine how far cancer has spread but can increase the risk of lymphedema.

- Post-op emotions can be intense and confusing: grief, relief, and fear often exist all at once.

- Lymphedema can develop weeks or even years later. Knowing early signs and daily prevention habits is crucial.

- Tumor grade (how aggressive) and stage (how far it's spread) help guide the treatment plan.

- Every stage matters. Every diagnosis deserves support, regardless of severity.

🤍 Key Takeaway

This chapter reminds us that healing is not linear. Even after surgery, there are setbacks, unknowns, and emotions to unpack. Your journey is valid no matter how it looks, and you're allowed to feel everything that comes with it.

"I just wanted to go through it quietly and privately, and I did."
—Edie Falco; Shared importance of privacy and self-care during recovery.

5
Oncology & Treatment Planning

After healing from surgery, it was time to meet with the oncologist. I can tell you that after my experience with the surgeon, I wasn't exactly skipping into this appointment with optimism and trust in the medical system. I was guarded, bracing myself for another round of being spoken *at* instead of *with*.

But this visit was different.

From the moment we arrived, something felt softer. More relaxed. My husband and I weren't stuck in a sterile waiting room under flickering fluorescent lights. We were immediately brought into *her actual office*. Carpeted floors, cozy chairs instead of that god-awful crinkly exam table. The lighting was soft, and it was the kind of atmosphere that made you exhale a little. There were family photos on her desk. Art on the walls. It felt more like a therapist's office than anything I'd seen in a hospital.

And then she walked in.

She had shoulder-length auburn curls and kind eyes. Her white lab coat was draped over a dress, and on her feet were pink sneakers. That detail struck me immediately. *Pink sneakers.* They told me everything I needed to know. She was grounded and real. She wasn't trying to impress anyone or stand behind some intimidating facade. I liked her instantly.

She looked me in the eye and asked how I was doing. Not like it was some box she had to check, either. It felt as though she genuinely wanted to know. It was the first time in weeks I felt seen. Actually seen. She didn't rush through her explanation or talk over our heads. She paused, often, to make sure we were following along. She answered the questions we had, and the ones we didn't even know to ask yet.

Then came the plan. Chemotherapy would be next. Because the tumor had been invasive and two lymph nodes were positive, we needed to be aggressive. I didn't fully understand the terminology, not yet. But I understood she cared. And because she cared, I trusted her.

Her compassion was the lifeline I was waiting for. A warm, sunny hug in the middle of an otherwise pitch-black storm. She treated me like a person, not just a case file. Not a random name on a list. She gave me options. She gave me time. She gave me *agency*. For the first time since hearing the words "you have cancer," I felt like I had even the tiniest bit of control.

If you're preparing to meet your oncologist, or maybe you already have, and you're sitting there overwhelmed and unsure, please, please hear me when I say this:

You deserve a care team that sees you.
Not just your bloodwork. Not just your scans. *You.*

Your emotions. Your voice. Your body. Your boundaries.

If you feel rushed, dismissed, or unheard, you have every right to ask more questions. You have every right to slow things down. Hell, if you still don't feel comfortable, you even have the right to say "thanks, but no thanks" and find someone who will treat you like a whole human being with thoughts and feelings.

One more time, louder, for those in the back of the room:

This is your life. Your fight. Your body.
And you deserve to feel safe and supported every step of the way.

Understanding Treatment Modalities

Therapy	Purpose	Common Side Effects
Chemotherapy	Kill rapidly dividing cells (neoadjuvant or adjuvant)	Hair loss, nausea, fatigue, low blood counts
Radiation Therapy	Destroy residual cells post-surgery	Skin irritation, fatigue, localized swelling
Hormone (Endocrine)	Block estrogen/ progesterone (ER/PR+)	Hot flashes, joint pain, bone density loss

Targeted Therapy	Attack specific proteins (e.g., HER2+)	Cardiac issues, diarrhea, fatigue
Immunotherapy	Boost immune response (e.g., PD-L1+)	Rash, thyroid dysfunction, fatigue

What Kind of Breast Cancer Do I Have?

When someone says they have "breast cancer," it sounds like one diagnosis. But really, it's a whole family of diseases with different names, behaviors, and treatment paths. Understanding what type of breast cancer you have helps shape everything that comes next.

Let's walk through the most common types.

◆ Invasive Ductal Carcinoma (IDC)

This is the most common type of breast cancer. "Invasive" means the cancer has spread beyond the milk ducts into nearby breast tissue. "Ductal" simply means it began in the milk ducts. IDC accounts for about 70–80% of all breast cancer diagnoses.

Rachele shared

"I was diagnosed with IDC, stage 2, with two positive lymph nodes. The moment I heard the word 'invasive,' I stopped listening. All I could think was, 'This thing is already on the move inside me.'"

Her words capture what many feel when they first hear that diagnosis. The fear. The urgency. But IDC is also highly treatable, especially when caught early and followed by a solid treatment plan.

◆ Invasive Lobular Carcinoma (ILC)

ILC begins in the lobules, the milk-producing glands, and spreads outward. It's the second most common type of breast cancer, making up 10–15% of cases. Unlike IDC, ILC tends to grow in a scattered or single-file pattern, which can make it harder to detect on mammograms.

Karen explained:

"Mine was ILC, and they didn't find it with the first mammogram. It was growing like a vine, not a lump. I knew something felt off, but everyone kept telling me things looked fine."

Her story reminds us how important it is to trust your instincts and advocate for follow-up when something doesn't feel right, even if the scan says otherwise. It's a reminder that we have to advocate for our own health when things don't seem quite right.

◆ Ductal Carcinoma In Situ (DCIS)

DCIS is considered "non-invasive." The abnormal cells are still confined to the milk ducts and haven't spread into surrounding breast tissue. It's sometimes called "stage 0." While it's not yet invasive cancer, it can become invasive if left untreated. DCIS is often highly treatable with surgery and possibly radiation.

◆ Lobular Carcinoma In Situ (LCIS)

LCIS is not technically cancer—it's a marker of increased risk. It means that abnormal cells have been found in the lobules, but they haven't spread. LCIS doesn't usually require immediate treatment, but it does mean you and your doctor will want to monitor things closely.

◆ Triple-Negative Breast Cancer (TNBC)

TNBC is defined by what it doesn't have. These tumors are negative for estrogen, progesterone, and HER2 receptors. Because of that, they don't respond to hormone therapies or HER2-targeted drugs.

Shanice recalled:

"Triple-negative. I had no idea what that meant, just that everyone's face got serious when they saw it. I learned quickly that it meant fewer options, but also, that I had to hit this hard and fast."

TNBC tends to be more aggressive and more likely to recur, especially in the first few years after treatment. But research is advancing rapidly, and many women respond very well to the current chemo and immunotherapy regimens.

◆ HER2-Positive Breast Cancer

This means the cancer cells are producing too much of a protein called HER2. These tumors tend to grow quickly, but they respond exceptionally well to targeted treatments like Herceptin or Perjeta. HER2-positive used to be one of the most aggressive subtypes, but it's also one of the biggest success stories in terms of treatment breakthroughs.

◆ Inflammatory Breast Cancer (IBC)

IBC is rare and aggressive. It doesn't usually form a lump. Instead, it may cause swelling, redness, or warmth in the breast, and is often mistaken for an infection.

Celeste shared:

Sharon tells us, "It looked like a rash. My breast was hot and red, and I kept being told it was an infection. It wasn't until the third doctor that someone said the word 'inflammatory.' I'd never even heard of that kind of breast cancer before."

IBC typically requires chemotherapy first to shrink the cancer before any surgery is done.

◆ Rare Subtypes (Metaplastic, etc.)

Some cancers, like Metaplastic Breast Cancer, are rare and behave very differently. These types may not respond to standard treatments and require more specialized care, sometimes involving clinical trials or second opinions from cancer centers with advanced expertise.

Yvette said, "I had Metaplastic carcinoma. Nobody around me had even heard of it. Every doctor appointment felt like I was entering unknown territory."

Being rare doesn't mean hopeless. Your journey might just require more tailored decisions.

🧬 Receptor Statuses

Each tumor is tested to find out what receptors it has. These are like keys that can help unlock the best treatment. Here's what they mean:

- **ER+ / PR+:** These tumors grow in response to estrogen or progesterone. Hormone-blocking therapies like Tamoxifen are often used.

- **HER2+:** These cancers overproduce a protein that speeds up growth. Targeted drugs like Herceptin stop it in its tracks.

- **Triple-Negative (ER-/PR-/HER2-):** These don't respond to hormone or HER2 drugs, so chemo and sometimes immunotherapy are used.

- **PD-L1+:** If present, immunotherapy may be an option to help the immune system recognize and destroy cancer cells.

Each of these markers helps answer: *What's driving the cancer? And how do we shut it down?*

☀ What is a Port-a-Cath?

If chemotherapy is part of your treatment plan, your oncologist might recommend having a port placed. Short for "port-a-cath," it's a small medical device that sits just under your skin, usually on the upper chest, and connects to one of the larger veins near your heart. It's about the size of a quarter, and once it's healed, it creates a little access point that makes getting IV medications, blood draws, and fluids much easier. This means no more needle hunts through your arm every time you walk in the door.

When my oncologist first brought it up, I wasn't so sure. I was already drowning in appointments, tests, and procedures, and the thought of yet another one felt like too much. Another incision? Another day under sedation? Hard pass. I'd already been through enough

72

But eventually, I agreed. And as I would soon learn, it turned out to be one of the best decisions I made during treatment.

The procedure itself was short and easy. I was sedated, and it took about an hour. I went home the same day with a bandage over the area and a mild soreness that faded after a few days. It left a small bump beneath the skin, something I could feel if I touched it, but otherwise, it wasn't noticeable. Once it healed, didn't really think about it much. What I did know was how much easier it made chemo days.

No anxious nurses prodding my arm like a pin cushion. No more collapsed veins or bruises from multiple sticks. With the port, each infusion was quicker, smoother, and a hell of a lot less stressful.

I'm not the only one who feels that way. Melanie told me, "My veins were awful. I'd end up in tears every time they tried to draw blood. The port changed everything. One little poke, and they were in. I wish I hadn't fought it so hard at first. It ended up being a godsend."

Carla said her nurses called it her "power button." She told me, "It made things easier. I didn't have to brace myself every time. And toward the end, it actually gave me comfort. Like, okay, I've done this before. I can do it again."

And then there's Tara, who put it simply but perfectly: "I was terrified of getting the port. But after the first chemo session, I realized it was the one thing that didn't hurt."

Ports do need a little TLC. Between treatments, they have to be flushed every few weeks to keep them from clotting, but the oncology nurses usually handle that during regular visits. After treatment ends, you don't have to rush to get it removed. Some people keep their port for months, just in case there's a need for more treatment, labs, or scans. I kept mine in for a full year after finishing chemo. Removing the port was a simple outpatient procedure, done with local anesthesia and very little downtime.

Looking back, I'm grateful I chose to get the port. It was one less thing to stress about in the middle of a very stressful season. If your doctor recommends one, ask your questions. Make sure you understand the process. But know this: for a lot of us, it's a small, barely visible bump that can make a big, visible difference in how treatment goes.

And if you're still on the fence about it, just imagine not having to explain your poor, overused arm veins to yet another nurse ever again. Worth it.

My Chemo Story

I remember my first chemo session clearly. They had me set up in a recliner, the IV line in my port, the fluorescent lights buzzing above me. Somewhere in the middle of the drip, the Benadryl they'd added to my cocktail kicked in and knocked me out cold. I slept while the medications did their work. After a bit, my husband looked over and saw that my face was bright red and flushed. I had spiked a 103°F fever, but didn't realize because I was asleep. Thankfully, he saw me and caught it. The nurse was able to respond quickly and adjust my dosage before things got worse.

That was just day one.

My chemo regimen was originally planned to last 48 weeks. But delays started showing up early. Some weeks, my bloodwork would come back showing my platelets had tanked too low for treatment. When that happened, they'd give me an injection, right into the soft fat of my stomach, that would kick my bone marrow into overdrive, urging it to produce more platelets. Once my counts bounced back, treatment would resume the following week.

This meant that what was supposed to be a 48-week cycle stretched out into nearly a full year. A year of weekly blood draws, lab results and sitting in infusion chairs. A year of needles and bruises and trying to convince myself, and everybody around me, that I was fine when I absolutely wasn't.

With time, my body learned the pattern. Tuesdays were chemo. By Wednesday, I'd start to crash. The fatigue would hit hard and heavy, and food would lose all appeal. That awful metallic taste would take over my mouth, like I had been sucking on nickels. I sleep a lot. I barely ate. The nausea and brain fog were constant companions.

By Friday afternoon, I'd rally just enough to drag myself back to work. I was bartending at the time, and in some strange way, the chaos helped. Making drinks, taking orders, pretending to be okay. It gave me a purpose, even when my body was screaming for rest. Over the weekends, I could almost pass for normal. I'd feel a little more like myself. And then Monday would arrive, and we'd start the whole damn thing over again.

As the weeks dragged into months, it got harder to show up. Harder to face that chair. Harder to let another needle slide into my skin. Harder to keep pretending that I was okay.

It also got harder to hear how "brave" I was. Harder to smile and nod while people told me how "strong" I was, how "inspiring." I knew they meant well. I knew they wanted to help and be encouraging. But their words started to feel like pressure. Like I wasn't allowed to be anything *but* strong. Like my pain needed to be palatable for everyone else.

So I told them I was fine. I smiled. I said I was "doing great." I kept their fear at bay by lying.

And worse, I was lying to myself, too.

🩺 Prepping for Treatment: Caring for Your Body Before the Storm

- **Nutrition:** Add fruits, veggies, proteins. Drink more water.
  Leah said: "Smoothies became a ritual. One thing I could control."

- **Movement:** Gentle walks or stretching help your body stay strong.
  Erica said: "Walking became sacred. It grounded me."

- **Sleep & Rest:** Prioritize winding down, even if sleep feels elusive.

- **Emotional Support:** Vanessa shared: "I didn't want to talk about how scared I was. Therapy helped me realize I didn't

75

have to be strong all the time."

- **Dental, Fertility & Medical:** Get a cleaning, discuss fertility if needed, and ask about vaccines or baseline heart tests.

- **Practical Prep:** Stock gentle foods. Create a chemo comfort kit.
Naomi said: "I made a 'cancer binder.' It sounds silly, but it gave me control."

Questions to Ask Your Oncologist

- What is the goal of treatment—curative or preventative?

- How long will treatment last? What are the phases?

- Will I need a port?

- What side effects should I expect?

- Are clinical trials an option?

- Is chemo the only path?

- What mental health or support services are available?

Chapter Highlights

- Your oncologist's compassion matters.

- Breast cancer has many subtypes—each with unique treatment paths.

- Knowing receptor status personalizes your plan.

- Ports can make chemo easier.

- Preparing your body, space, and emotions helps ease the overwhelm.

- You have the right to ask questions and make decisions that feel right for you.

🤍 Key Takeaway

This chapter is about reclaiming your power—not by knowing everything, but by asking, listening, and showing up for yourself. When your medical team treats you with humanity and respect, it restores your faith in the process. And when *you* treat yourself with kindness and care, it becomes the foundation for everything that comes next.

"Hair is overrated."
—Melissa Etheridge; Encouraged self-exams;
Normalized chemo hair loss by appearing bald at the Grammys

6
What They Don't Tell You About Radiation Therapy

After nearly a year of chemo, I can assure you, there were plenty of days when I didn't want to go. I was tired, mentally and physically. But somehow, each week, I kept showing up.

But radiation is what finally broke me.

When we first talked about it, it sounded so simple. The appointments would only take about 30 minutes. Five days a week. In and out. No big deal. I remember thinking, *Easy-peasy*. I'd had sunburns before. I figured maybe it would sting a little, maybe make me tired, but nothing I couldn't handle.

But radiation doesn't hit you like a truck. It's not one dramatic blow. It's a slow, steady unraveling. It creeps in so quietly that you don't even realize it at first. And then, one morning, you wake up and realize that you're held together by thread. And that thread is fraying fast.

Somewhere around the halfway mark, I hit the wall. A thick, heavy, unmoving wall that I couldn't climb over or crawl under. My body ached. My emotions were shot. I was tired in a way that sleep couldn't touch. It was a bone-deep, soul-level tired. And I couldn't keep on pretending that I was okay.

So, I took a break.

There were a lot of factors behind that decision, and I go into more detail in the mental health chapter. But I'll say this: stepping back was the right call for me. I needed that break. Not just to let my body rest, but to start untangling the emotional knots I'd been carrying around since the day I heard the word "cancer." I was too tired to keep pretending everything was okay.

Then there was the stillness. The absolute stillness. During each session, I'd lie still on the table. There was no music, no talking, just the mechanical hum of the machine. I wasn't there long enough to fall asleep. I was there just long enough for my thoughts to start screaming. And they did. Everything I had pushed down came bubbling up to the surface. The fear. The grief. The unraveling of a marriage that had been barely holding together since diagnosis. The deep, aching loneliness of living under the same roof with someone who felt more like a roommate than a partner.

Somewhere between week three and week five, I realized I couldn't keep pretending. I couldn't keep showing up for everyone else if I didn't first show up for myself. I was at my breaking point, and I wasn't alone.

Julie, another survivor, said it like this, "Radiation therapy was more mentally exhausting than anything else I had faced. I dreaded the silence. Just me and the machine and my thoughts. It forced me to deal with things I had pushed aside for months."

Radiation affects everyone differently. Some people breeze through with minor skin irritation and a little fatigue. Others, like me, walk away with invisible bruises. It wasn't my skin that burned the most. It was my spirit.

Ellie shared something that echoed my own truth, "The radiation burns on my skin were nothing compared to the way it burned through my spirit. I felt like I lost myself for a while there. But every time I made it to my appointment, I reminded myself, I'm still showing up."

And sometimes, the only things that really kept me going were the smallest, most unexpected moments of grace.

One day, after a session, the radiation tech smiled at me and said, "Did you know that you wiggle your toes the entire time you're in there?" I didn't. I had no idea, but it made me laugh. And now, even years later, I catch myself wiggling my toes whenever I'm overwhelmed. It's like my body found its own little way to soothe me when everything else felt out of control.

So if you're in the thick of it right now, and you're exhausted, and you're wondering how the hell you're going to keep doing this, I want you to hear this loud and clear:

You are not weak. Keep going. You are not failing. And you are not alone.

You are a survivor. A warrior. And *real* healing requires so much more than just medicine. It takes space., rest., and plenty of grace.
Oh… and the radical, defiant decision to keep showing up, even when it hurts like hell.

What to Expect from Radiation Therapy

Radiation uses focused, high-energy beams to kill off any remaining cancer cells after surgery. It's most common after a lumpectomy or if lymph nodes were involved. You may not feel anything while it's happening, but the impact builds over time. It's usually done five days a week, for anywhere between four and eight weeks. Each session takes about 10 to 20 minutes, but don't be surprised if it leaves you drained for hours afterward. Some people even need medical breaks mid-treatment, and that's okay. Speak up and ask.

During the session itself, you lie down on a table while a machine rotates around your body. The machine doesn't touch you, and the beams are invisible. You don't feel them in the moment. But over time, skin irritation and fatigue tend to creep in. And there is the mental toll that often lands hardest in the quiet after.

Physical & Emotional Side Effects

The side effects of radiation are wildly unpredictable. Two people can go through identical treatment plans: same dosage, same schedule, same machine, and walk away with completely different experiences. For some, it's just a little skin irritation. A mild redness, maybe a bit of tenderness. For others, it's burns that peel and sting and make wearing a bra or even a shirt feel like dragging sandpaper across raw nerves.

And then of course the fatigue.
It doesn't always hit right away. It sneaks in slowly, wrapping itself around your bones until even getting off the couch feels like climbing

Everest. You'll think you're doing fine, and then one day, your body simply won't cooperate. You'll need naps you didn't used to take. Your limbs will feel heavy. You'll start forgetting what it ever felt like to not be tired.

But what really throws people off, is how emotional the aftermath can be.

Sometimes, you feel okay at first. You get through your sessions. You check the boxes. You ring the bell. But weeks later, something shifts. Maybe your chest tightens every time you raise your arm. Maybe you find yourself staring at the ceiling at 3 a.m. because your body won't fully relax. Maybe the grief hits out of nowhere; the grief you didn't have time to deal with because chemo had you stuck in survival mode.

Tamika, a fellow survivor, said it perfectly, "Everyone said radiation would be easy. But I hit week five and couldn't stop crying. I wasn't even sure why. I think it was just everything finally catching up to me. It wasn't the treatment. It was the weight of all I had survived."

"Radiation was sneaky. I thought I was fine until week four," Camilla said. "I hit a wall emotionally."

"They told me about skin burn," Jason shared, "but they didn't tell me how tired I'd be. Like bone-tired."

And Dana added, "Stretching helped. I didn't want to move at first, but it gave me back control over my body."

Some survivors found unexpected clarity during radiation. One woman told me she used those silent minutes to thank her body for surviving, again and again. Another said lying still each day became a quiet ritual, a sacred moment where she finally stopped running and just *was*.

Radiation may not be as flashy or dramatic as chemo, but don't underestimate it. It chips away at you slowly, and sometimes, gently, but it gets under your skin in ways you don't expect.

So if you're in that space now, feeling confused or tired or undone, please know you're not broken. This part of the journey can be just as demanding as everything that came before it. The wounds it leaves aren't always visible—but that doesn't make them any less real.

Give yourself grace.

Grieve, stretch, cry, rest, rage. Do what your body and spirit need.

You're still here. And that matters more than anything.

Common Physical Side Effects of Radiation Therapy

Timing	Side Effect	Tips & Tools That Help
Short-Term (During or Soon After	Skin burns, peeling, or redness (like a sunburn)	Use doctor-approved creams, avoid tight clothing, let skin breathe
	Fatigue that builds slowly and lasts all	Prioritize rest, listen to your body, hydrate, keep a light
	Irritation or sensitivity in the	Avoid underwire bras, wear loose cotton clothing, ask
	Emotional exhaustion, especially	Give yourself grace, talk with a therapist or support group,
Medium-Term (1–6 Months Post-	Lingering fatigue or "body heaviness"	Gentle movement, rest as needed, consider short naps or stretching routines
	Tightness or restricted motion in	Try physical therapy, daily stretching, warm compresses
	Difficulty sleeping or relaxing due to	Experiment with pillows for support, use calming
	Emotional flatness or delayed grief	Journaling, therapy, allow feelings to come when
Long-Term (6 Months – Years Later)	Fibrosis (thickening or scarring of tissue)	Long-term physical therapy, massage therapy, communicate with your
	Sensitivity or tenderness in the	Wear soft fabrics, avoid pressure, manage discomfort
	Uneven texture or firmness in the chest	Understand it's normal, consider gentle massage,
	Body image struggles due to asymmetry or	Seek support groups, allow space for grief, explore

Post-Treatment Recovery & Scar Care

Radiation doesn't just stop when the machine does. The effects linger, and can sometimes last for months. Gentle movement helps. So does moisturizing daily with fragrance-free lotions. If your skin feels tight, or your range of motion changes, ask about physical therapy, especially with someone that specializes in oncology recovery. Manual lymphatic drainage can help with swelling and tenderness.

Start with slow stretching, and build up as you feel ready. There's no race to the finish line here. Take your time and go slow. Progress is progress, no matter how small.

Questions Worth Asking Your Care Team

- Are there specific skin care products you recommend?

- What signs should I watch for when it comes to fibrosis or complications?

- Should I be doing stretches or movement exercises now—or later?

- How will we monitor healing over time?

- What emotional health support is available during or after radiation?

FAQ: Living Life While in Radiation

Q: When do side effects usually start?
A: Most people begin to feel them around weeks 2–3. Fatigue may persist for a few weeks after treatment ends.

Q: What helps with emotional burnout?
A: Don't keep it all inside. Talk early and often. Let someone hold space for you. You don't have to be strong every minute.

✅ Chapter Highlights

- Radiation may seem like the "easy" part of cancer treatment, but its toll, especially emotionally, builds quietly.

- No two people experience it the same. There is no "right" or "wrong" reaction.

- Fatigue, grief, skin irritation, and emotional collapse are all valid responses.

- The treatment may be silent, but it's far from still. It forces a kind of reckoning; one that can bring clarity or pain or both.

🩶 Key Takeaway

This chapter isn't only about what radiation does to your body. It's about what it does to your soul. If you find yourself falling apart halfway through or crying in the car after a session, please know that what you are doing is hard. And you are doing it anyway.

And that is the very definition of brave.

"Just because someone is young doesn't mean they can't get breast cancer."
—*Kylie Minogue; urged younger women to pay attention to symptoms despite age stereotypes*

7

Managing the Side Effects

I remember the day my oncologist gave us the list. It was like something you'd get from the pharmacy with a new prescription, except this wasn't for just one medication. It was a whole stack of possibilities, layered with medical terms and percentages. A list of everything that could happen once chemo started. Short-term effects. Long-term effects. It was a lot to process.

That night, my husband and I sat at the kitchen table, both of us staring at that paper like it had fangs. Nausea. Fatigue. Mouth sores. Neuropathy. Brain fog. Bone pain. Heart damage. Fertility loss. Hair loss. Kidney disease. The words blurred together, but the message was clear: this is going to suck.

And then came the question, the one no one wants to say out loud, but every one of us thinks at some point: *Is it worth putting my body through all of it?*

The surgeon had already removed the tumor. Maybe that was enough. Have we exhausted all other options? What if there was something else we could try that wouldn't wreck my body in the process. This felt like too much. Maybe I wasn't strong enough to survive it. Would our marriage survive it?

We took all those fears, every last one of them, back to my oncologist. We laid out all of our concerns. And to her credit, she didn't brush us off. She didn't guilt us or rush us. She listened to our concerns. She really *heard* us. And then she told us something that changed everything.

She said we weren't locking ourselves into anything. That I'd be monitored constantly with weekly bloodwork, regular heart scans, open conversations at every step. If something didn't feel right, if it got too hard, or if my body started to wave the white flag, we could reassess. We could shift the plan. We could pivot.

That reassurance really did help me feel better about moving forward with her plan.

I didn't want to feel like I was signing up for suffering just to check a box. I needed to know that someone would walk this with me. That I wouldn't be left to navigate it on my own if things got bad. And in that moment, I felt like my doctor was in my corner. It made all the difference in the world to me.

Still... even with that reassurance, the side effects came. Some I expected. Some completely blindsided me. And no list, no matter how thorough or well-intentioned, can truly prepare you for what it feels like to live in a body going through chemotherapy.

So if you're sitting here, reading this and wondering how the hell you're supposed to do this, let me say something loud and clear: **If it gets really hard, that doesn't mean you're failing.** Fighting cancer is a full-time job. Nobody else can clock in and do this for you. We have to pull up our Big Girl Panties and participate, even when we don't want to. Especially when we don't want to.

But if you ever hit that point where your gut is screaming, *"I can't keep doing this,"* don't ignore it. Don't try to tough it out alone. Talk to your oncologist and see if there's another way. Ask the uncomfortable questions and look at every option to figure out what your next step needs to be for *you*.

This is about getting through it in a way that's survivable.

You've got this. I promise **you're stronger than you think.** And if you ever forget it, I'm here to remind you.

What follows is a chart of chemo side effects. These are some of the most common things people experience, and some of the ways that helped me, and others, get through them. Keep in mind that everyone is different, though. You might not deal with all of them. Or, you might have ones that aren't even listed here.

Let's take it one symptom, one day, one deep breath at a time.

Managing Side Effects

Side Effect	When It Might Occur	Tips & Tools That Help
Nausea	Day of and after chemo	Antiemetics, small meals, ginger chews or tea
Hair loss	As early as 2–3 weeks after first treatment	Shave early to reduce emotional impact; try scarves, wigs
Fatigue	Midweek during chemo cycles	Plan rest days, hydrate, gentle movement
Metallic taste	During/after infusion	Use plastic utensils, avoid favorite foods
Low immunity	Ongoing	Wash hands, avoid crowds, stay up-to-date on labs
Constipation/ Hemorrhoids	First few days after chemo or anti-nausea meds	Stay hydrated, eat fiber-rich foods, ask doctor about stool softeners
Mouth sores	A few days after chemo starts	Rinse with baking soda/salt water, avoid spicy/acidic foods, use a soft toothbrush
Nosebleeds	Randomly during treatment (due to dryness)	Use a humidifier, apply nasal saline spray, avoid nose blowing or picking
Bone Pain	Randomly	Heating pads, Claritin
Appetite changes	Ongoing or cyclical	Eat small, frequent meals, try new textures/flavors, don't force favorite foods
Diarrhea	During or after chemo, varies by drug	Stay hydrated, avoid dairy and high-fiber foods, ask doctor about medications
Skin changes/ Acne	Ongoing	Use gentle moisturizers, avoid fragranced products, sun protection is essential

Nail changes	Weeks into treatment	Keep nails short, avoid polish/remover, use thick hand creams
Peripheral neuropathy	Weeks into chemo or later	Report to your care team, avoid extreme temperatures, wear comfy shoes and gloves
Sleep disturbances	Anytime during treatment	Maintain a routine, avoid caffeine late in the day, ask about safe sleep aids
Weight gain or loss	Gradual	Track eating gently, move when you can, ask for a dietitian referral

✎ Tara C., Diagnosed at 46

I found the lump in the middle of the night. It was small, but something in me just knew. I had no family history, no major risk factors, and yet within weeks, I was hearing the word "cancer." What was first believed to be Stage 0 turned out to be Stage 2B invasive breast cancer with lymph node involvement. That one small mass carried far more weight than any of us expected.

Chemo was brutal. Every part of me hurt, even my fingernails. My tongue stuck to the roof of my mouth from how dry it was. My nose bled. My back ached. I couldn't sleep, yet my body felt too heavy to move. Nausea twisted through my stomach, but I couldn't go to the bathroom. Every inch of me felt like it was breaking down, and I couldn't tell if it was the medicine or the fear that made it worse. I remember thinking more than once, "I don't know if I can do this again."

Oddly enough, when I could move, I played hockey. For about a week after each infusion, I was completely down. But if I had even a shred of strength before the next round, I laced up and played. It didn't make the pain go away, but it reminded me I was still in there somewhere.

Radiation came next. Sixteen rounds. By the end, I had third-degree burns across my chest. The pain was sharp, constant, and raw. I used cheesecloth soaked in thick cream three times a day, wrapping it like armor. It helped, a little. But the sting of radiation lasted long after the final session.

People don't talk about how expensive the side effects are. The anti-nausea meds, the constipation relief, the burn creams. It adds up. And the emotional cost is even higher.

Through it all, I stayed close to my family and tried to lean on my friends, but unless someone has been through it, they can't truly understand. Not the pain. Not the fear. Not the exhaustion that lives in your bones.

I'm still here. I'm still healing. But the memory of chemo doesn't fade easily. It lives in the background, a quiet reminder of just how hard I had to fight to stay standing.

Oh, The Hair

No matter how much you think you know about chemo and hair loss, chances are you're still not emotionally prepared for the day your hair starts falling out in clumps. For me, it was like someone flipped a switch while I was sleeping. I woke up one day and it was coming out by the handfuls. I was shocked!

I've never been a vain person, so beforehand, I didn't think it would be a very big deal. I knew it was coming and I felt prepared for it. But it was a big deal. It felt like a *very* big deal. By this point, my emotions were already so raw, so shredded, that I just didn't have the capacity for *one more thing*.

My girls were home from school that day, so I spent most of it hiding in the shower. I didn't want to scare them with my tears or have them see just how broken I felt. The motherly instinct to protect them at all cost was still there. So I just kept getting locking the bathroom door and getting into the shower, over and over, sobbing until I ran out of hot water, just trying to hold myself together while everything else was falling apart.

That evening, when my husband got home, we went to dinner with friends. We all talked about what was happening, and I decided I couldn't just let my hair fall out. I asked my husband to shave my head. I needed to take control of *something*.

We were in our friend's garage, with our oldest daughter sitting on my lap, arms wrapped around me, while the clippers buzzed and we cried together. Then, without hesitation, my husband shaved his head too. And his friend. These big, grown men, standing there with clumps of their hair on the floor, mingled withy own, giving me this quiet, beautiful moment of solidarity. It was such an emotional evening, but I'll always believe we handled it the best way we knew how; together.

Eventually, I lost it all. Not just the hair on my head, but every last strand. Arms, legs, underarms. Even the little peach fuzz we don't talk about. The only survivors were a few lashes and some stubborn eyebrows, but even those thinned out over time. My brows never really came back the same. To this day, I still color in their patchiness on most mornings. It's practically muscle memory by now.

But the hair on my head surprised me in the best way. When it grew back, it came in thicker. Prettier. Curlier. I didn't expect to love it, but I did. Somehow, it felt like a reward. Like this small, unexpected gift after everything my body had endured. A soft, wild crown that whispered, *you're healing*.

For some people, the answer is to get a wig that they like. I had a couple, but rarely wore them. Baldness and cancer didn't stop me from going to Daytona Bike Week that year on the back of my husband's motorcycle. That first day, I wore the cutest wig you've ever seen, braided it into pigtails. I looked adorable. But between the Florida heat and my damn helmet, I was roasting. That thing was itchy, sweaty, and just *not it*.

So the next day, I said screw it. I threw on a bandanna and went about my day. Eventually, I yanked that off too and walked around bald, head shining like a cue ball in the sun, and I didn't give a damn.

Now, if you've never spent time in the biker community, you might think it's all leather and growls and tough guys who'd rather ride through a wall than talk about feelings. But let me tell that those people have some of the biggest hearts I've ever known. I got more hugs that day than I could count. I heard story after story from these big, burly men about their moms, sisters, wives… all survivors. Fighters. Women they loved. Women who lived. They shared their pain, their victories, their hope. With *me*, a stranger.

92

And I'll never forget it.

That experience changed something in me. I walked around bald and instead of shame, I felt power. That bald head of mine became a symbol. A battle flag. And the community I found that day reminded me that I wasn't alone. That even in the middle of something so dark, there were people who would stand beside me, even if just for a moment.

So if you're standing in front of the mirror, holding back tears as you watch your hair fall away, just remember this: it's okay to grieve. It's okay to cry. But don't let it convince you that you've lost yourself.

Because the day will come when soft fuzz starts to grow. And when it does, a new version of you will begin to emerge like a butterfly. And she's beautiful as hell.

Cold Capping: A Glimmer of Control

Hair loss can feel like one of the most emotionally painful parts of chemotherapy. For some, it's the moment when the world can finally see what's happening inside their body. Cold capping, also known as scalp cooling, is a technique that offers a bit of control in an otherwise uncontrollable time. The process involves wearing a very cold cap before, during, and after chemo to reduce blood flow to the scalp. This helps limit how much of the chemo drugs reach your hair follicles, which can reduce or even prevent hair loss. It doesn't work for everyone, and it isn't compatible with all chemo regimens, but many women have found it to be a lifeline for their self-esteem. Cold capping is time-consuming, sometimes expensive, and can cause headaches or discomfort, but for those who choose it, it can feel like one thing they get to say "yes" to. One thing they get to keep. If it's something you're considering, talk with your oncologist to see if it's a safe option for you.

When Everything Tastes Like Metal

One of the weirdest things about chemo is how it hijacks your taste buds.

Suddenly, your favorite foods taste wrong. Water tastes like pennies. Even your mouth might feel coated in something bitter or sour that won't go away. This metallic or chemical taste, called **dysgeusia,** is a common side effect of chemotherapy and certain medications. It can last for weeks or even months, and for many survivors, it's one of the most frustrating changes to deal with.

You're not imagining it, and no, you're not being picky.
Your mouth really *has* changed.

What causes it?

Chemo affects the rapidly dividing cells in your body, including the cells in your mouth and taste buds. It can also change how your brain interprets smell, which also affects how things taste. Medications like cisplatin, carboplatin, doxorubicin, and cyclophosphamide are especially known for causing this.

What Can Help

Try these gentle tricks to make eating more tolerable, and maybe even enjoyable again:

- **Switch to plastic or bamboo utensils.**
  Metal silverware can make the metallic taste worse.

- **Use tart flavors to cut through the bitterness.**
  Lemon, lime, vinegar, pickles, green apples, or a splash of citrus in water can help neutralize the taste.

- **Rinse before eating.**
  A saltwater or baking soda mouth rinse (1/4 tsp salt + 1/4 tsp baking soda in 1 cup warm water) can help reset your mouth before meals.

- **Marinate or season food generously.**
  Herbs, garlic, onion, mustard, and bold spices like curry or chili can overpower unpleasant tastes. But be cautious if your mouth is sore. Avoid hot or acidic things in that case.

- **Stay away from red meat if it tastes "off."**
  Some people find red meat gets a strong metallic taste. Chicken, eggs, tofu, or beans may be more tolerable.

- **Suck on hard candy or mints.**
  Ginger chews, lemon drops, or sugar-free peppermint can refresh your mouth and improve appetite.

- **Try cold or room-temperature foods.**
  Hot foods release more aroma, which can amplify strange tastes. Smoothies, yogurts, fruit bowls, or chilled pasta salad might go down easier.

- **Hydrate often, but try flavored water if plain water tastes bad.**
  Add a splash of fruit juice, cucumber, mint, or ginger. Even coconut water or low-sugar electrolyte drinks can help if water feels too metallic.

- **Keep experimenting.**
  What works one day might not work the next. That's okay. The goal is to keep trying without judging yourself.

"It felt like I was chewing on nickels every time I tried to eat," one survivor told me. "Lemon water was my lifesaver. I kept a pitcher in the fridge every day."

The important thing is making sure your body is getting nourishment, and feeling somewhat normal in the middle of something super abnormal. You deserve food that comforts you, that fuels you, and that doesn't make you gag.

This will get better. It won't last forever, and your taste buds will heal. But until then, keep going gently, one bite at a time.

⚖ The Weight No One Warned Me About

I blew up like a balloon from the steroids they gave me during chemo. It was like waking up in someone else's body. I was slower, puffier, and felt totally unrecognizable. The scale started creeping up, my face looked like it had been inflated with a damn bike pump, and my clothes were suddenly conspiring against me. I knew it was from the meds. They warned me about fatigue, hair loss, and nausea, but no one pulled me aside to say, "Oh, by the way, your pants might stop fitting and your self-esteem might take a nosedive."

No one told me how hard it would be to lose that weight afterward.

I wasn't some couch potato before all this. I grew up a farm kid, throwing hay bales, mucking stalls, and hauling five-gallon buckets of water. Later, I joined the Navy, where I discovered my love for lifting weights and crushing PT. I was strong. The kind of strong that comes from grit and sweat and showing up. I took pride in my body and what it could do. But cancer had other plans.

During treatment, I didn't feel strong. I felt sick. I felt swollen. I felt too broken to move, let alone work out. The weight gain hit hard, not just physically, but emotionally. No one warned me how betrayed I would feel by the body I had once trusted to do anything I asked of it.

Weight gain during and after treatment is incredibly common, and yet it's one of those side effects people rarely mention. For many of us, the number on the scale isn't tied to what we're eating or how often we move, but to what our bodies have been through. The medications, steroids, hormone blockers, the forced estrogen crash... all of it throws your system out of whack. Your metabolism slows to a crawl, and your body holds on to every calorie like it's facing a harsh winter.

Your body doesn't feel like yours anymore. It's foreign. Your joints ache. The energy's gone. Your digestion is weird. You might be too tired to cook, let alone meal prep. And on top of it all, the weight just... hangs on.

And don't even get me started on the emotional toll. You look in the mirror and see the physical cost of survival. The puffiness. The bloating. The soft, unfamiliar curves. Your body has been through hell, and now it's trying to protect you in the only way it knows how; by holding onto every ounce of energy it can. That doesn't make it easier to accept, though. You're carrying grief and anger and trauma, all wrapped up in this new body that doesn't quite feel like home.

And unfortunately, conventional diets don't always work for us. You can cut carbs, track points, sip green sludge, and follow every sparkly Instagram coach who promises a 30-day miracle, and your body still might say, "Nope, we're good right here, thanks."

Everything has changed. Your hormones are doing the tango. Your cortisol is through the roof. Your sleep is trash. Your gut is still trying to remember what "normal" even felt like. And underneath all of it is the truth that your body isn't just carrying weight, but is also carrying all that trauma.

You're not lazy. You're not doing it wrong. Your body is just trying to recover from something big, and it needs compassion more than criticism.

So if you're standing in your closet wondering why nothing fits, or feeling betrayed by your own reflection, I see you. You are not lazy. You are not broken. You are recovering from the fight of your life.

And maybe the first step isn't jumping into a diet. Maybe it's placing your hand on your belly and saying, "Thank you for getting me through." Maybe it's finding gentle ways to move your body that don't feel like punishment. Maybe it's rest. Maybe it's grace. Maybe it's just making peace with the fact that your body is still figuring things out.

So what *does* help?

   Start with compassion. You didn't fail. Your body didn't betray you. It did what it had to do to survive.

   Focus on nourishment, not restriction. Choose foods that help reduce inflammation, like whole grains, leafy greens, berries, beans, lean protein, and healthy fats. Focus on what to add, not just what to cut.

   Move your body, gently and consistently. Strength training can help rebuild muscle mass lost during treatment. Even walking, yoga, and swimming make a difference. The goal isn't punishment, it's reconnecting with your body in ways that feel good. Don't overdo it.

Balance your blood sugar. Many survivors are more insulin-resistant post-treatment. Smaller, protein-rich meals throughout the day can help avoid blood sugar crashes and reduce cravings.

Check in with your medical team. Sometimes hormone blockers cause thyroid shifts or other metabolic issues. Ask for bloodwork. Advocate for yourself if something feels off.

Sleep matters. Deep, consistent rest can lower cortisol, improve hunger hormones, and support healing. And let's be honest, no one makes great choices when they're exhausted.

Consider working with a specialist. An oncology-informed dietitian or functional medicine practitioner can tailor a plan that actually works for *you*, not the version of you from before cancer.

Most importantly: **Give yourself time.**

This weight didn't appear overnight, and it won't leave overnight either. It will take compassion, community, and a whole lot of grace.

The Joint and Bone Pain

This one caught me completely off guard.

I wasn't expecting the kind of deep, aching pain that settled into my hips and legs during treatment. It wasn't just soreness, it sat in my bones. At first, I was convinced something was seriously wrong. I thought, "Great. Is it spreading? Is this a new nightmare starting?" But no, it turns out bone pain is a *very* common side effect, especially if you're getting injections like **Neulasta** or **Neupogen**, which are used to boost your white blood cell count after chemo.

These meds work by kickstarting your bone marrow into overdrive. They tell your body, "Hey, we need more cells and we need them now," and your bone marrow, bless it, gets to work like a panicked factory on the night shift. Problem is, when your marrow is cranking out new cells like that, you can *feel it.*

For me, it felt a lot like those "growing pains" I had as a kid, but worse. It was deeper, more intense, and harder to shake. There were nights when I curled up under a heated blanket with tears in my eyes, just waiting for it to pass. And it didn't pass quickly. Some days, it felt like my skeleton had its own separate, miserable personality.

And here's something I *really* wish I had known:
Claritin. Yes, the over-the-counter allergy medication. Sounds ridiculous, right? But it's actually often recommended by oncologists to help manage bone pain from white blood cell boosters. Something in the way it moderates inflammation seems to take the edge off. Some people swear by it. I didn't find out until *much* later, so I don't have any personal experience with it, but I wish someone had told me. As always, ask your doctor first, because every body is different, and you want to make sure it's safe for your specific case.

Also, bone and joint pain isn't just a short-term thing. If you're on **hormone therapy** like **tamoxifen** or **aromatase inhibitors**, that discomfort might hang around or even pop up months down the line. These meds can mess with your estrogen, which plays a huge role in bone density. That can lead to stiffness, aching joints, or even a kind of low-level pain that just never quite leaves. It's not all in your head. You're not being dramatic. These side effects are real, and they deserve to be addressed.

If you're feeling a weird pressure in your bones, an ache that just won't quit, or a general sense that your skeleton is staging a quiet rebellion, talk to your care team. Don't brush it off. Don't convince yourself it's just something you have to live with.

Pain is pain. And just because it's "common" doesn't mean it's normal. Or that you should suffer in silence.

Low Platelets & Bleeding Risks:

- **Why It Happens:** Chemotherapy can reduce platelet counts, increasing bleeding risk.

- **Signs:** Frequent nosebleeds, easy bruising, or bleeding from small cuts. For me, even leaning forward to get out of bed could sometimes trigger a nosebleed.

- **Prevention & Care:**
  - Keep a humidifier in your bedroom to prevent dry nasal passages.
  - Avoid blowing your nose hard; pinch the soft part of your nose gently and lean forward to stop bleeding.
  - Use a soft toothbrush and electric razor to minimize cuts.
  - Report persistent or heavy bleeding to your care team; they may prescribe platelet-boosting injections or transfusions.

Tracking Tip: Log any bleeding episodes in a journal or take notes on your phone, to discuss platelet management with your doctor.

Periodic Monitoring & Flexibility

Additional imaging scans or blood tests may be performed during treatment to monitor progress, assess response, and detect potential side effects. Common monitoring tests include:

Complete Blood Count (CBC): Weekly or before each chemotherapy session to check white blood cells, red blood cells, and platelets.

Liver & Kidney Function Panels: Blood tests to ensure organs can process and clear medications safely.

MUGA Scan (Multigated Acquisition Scan): A nuclear imaging test to evaluate heart ejection fraction, often used to monitor potential chemotherapy-related cardiotoxicity.

Echocardiogram: An ultrasound of the heart to visualize structure and function, sometimes used alongside MUGA.

Tumor Marker Tests (e.g., CA 15-3, CEA): Blood tests that may help track disease activity in certain types of breast cancer.

Bone Density Scan (DEXA): To assess bone health before or after hormone therapies that can affect bone density.

🌫 Chemo Brain: Your Thoughts Feel Fuzzy

If you've ever walked into a room and forgotten why, lost your train of thought mid-sentence, or sat there and stared at a familiar word until it looked made up, welcome to the club. This foggy, slow-motion mental state is lovingly referred to as "chemo brain," and while that name makes it sound kind of cute, like it might come with a fuzzy pink hat and a matching tote bag, it's anything but. It's frustrating, and it can feel like you've been handed someone else's brain with zero warning and no return policy.

For many people, chemo brain shows up as forgetting appointments, names, or entire conversations. Losing your words mid-thought or mid-sentence. Difficulty focusing, especially when multitasking. That constant feeling that your brain is buffering like a bad internet connection.

And let's be clear. This isn't "just in your head." (Well, I mean, technically it is, but not in the gas-lighty way people tend to imply.) Studies have shown that cancer treatment, including chemo, radiation, hormone therapy, anesthesia, and even just the all-consuming stress of diagnosis, can impact brain function. Your body is fighting a war. Of course your brain is tired. It's trying to keep you alive. That requires bandwidth.

Before cancer, I was sharp. I could tell you where anything was in the house, even if it hadn't seen daylight in six years. I remembered birthdays, science facts, phone numbers, and where the damn remote was. I could do math in my head without breaking a sweat and tell you which drawer your favorite hoodie was in, without even having to look.

I wasn't a genius. But I was clear. Quick. Confident.

And then I had cancer.

I finished chemo in 2008, and I swear to you, there was a line. Before chemo, I was fine. After chemo, I wasn't. Something shifted, and my brain never bounced back.

Now I lose things constantly. I put the peanut butter in the bathroom and the toothpaste in the pantry. My husband recently got me an AirTag for my keys because I kept losing them. I walk into a room and forget what I came in for. I mix up my kid's names with the dog's names. Sometimes I'll be talking and mid-sentence "poof" the words are gone. Words I know that I know. They just vanish like smoke. And when they do finally come back, I'm already five thoughts behind and completely lost in the conversation.

Kristie told me about the time she blanked on her own ZIP code at the pharmacy. "It was like my brain just unplugged itself," she said. "The pharmacist looked at me like I was high. I wanted to scream, 'I'm not stupid, I'm just on chemo!'"
I nodded so hard when I read that, I gave myself a headache. It's not forgetfulness. It's disorientation. It's being betrayed by your own mind in front of other people and trying not to fall apart.

And it's not just inconvenient. It's humiliating. It makes you feel broken in ways you never expected. I grieve the brain I used to have. And no, this isn't "just getting older." People try to relate, "Oh, I do that too! It's just aging!" but I was 31. Not 75. I didn't have brain fog before chemo. There was a clear difference.

Arlene described it perfectly. "Chemo brain made me feel like a ghost in my own life. I'd walk into a room and forget why I was there. Or stare at a familiar face and not remember their name. It was like I was fading, piece by piece."
That line crushed me. Because it's not just losing track of your thoughts, it's losing pieces of yourself and wondering if you'll ever get them back.

If I had to describe it, I'd say it's like trying to read without your glasses. You know the words are there, but they're blurry. You have to squint, tilt your head, maybe blink a few times to make sense of things. It's not impossible. But it's a hell of a lot harder. And it's exhausting.

Monica said what so many of us feel but don't expect: "People warned me about the nausea and the fatigue, but no one prepared me for the brain fog. I was in the middle of telling a story and just... lost it. My daughter had to finish my sentence. That shook me more than anything."

We brace ourselves for the physical toll, but the mental toll sneaks in and stays longer than we thought it would.

That's what my brain feels like now.

It doesn't mean I'm not smart anymore. But it does mean that everything takes more effort. More concentration. More patience. From me, and from the people around me. And the worst part is that sometimes I can feel the judgment. The sigh. The barely concealed irritation from someone who thinks I'm being slow, or forgetful, or careless.

But I'm not. I'm doing the best I can with the brain I've got now.

Chemo brain is real. It's not an excuse. It's not laziness. It's not "just stress." It is a cost I paid to stay alive. And while I'm immensely grateful to still be here, I also mourn the sharpness I lost. Both things can be true. Gratitude and grief can live in the same breath.

What Helps

Lists are lifesavers
I call myself the "Sticky Note Queen." Use sticky notes, to-do apps, voice memos, whatever works for you. Write things down before you forget, even if it's just "remember to eat lunch."

Use your phone for reminders
Set alarms for medications, appointments, hydration, and rest. Let your phone carry some of the mental load. I use my phone to remind me to feed our fish each day, because I tend to get busy and forget.

Do one thing at a time
Multitasking becomes nearly impossible when your brain is fogged. That's okay. Focus on one task, then finish it and move on. If I don't do this, I'll have 20 things started and nothing finished.

Rest your mind, not just your body
Mental fatigue is real. Breaks, deep breathing, meditation, even a good cry can give your brain a much-needed pause.

Tell people what's going on

You don't have to pretend everything's fine. Let friends and family know you're struggling with chemo brain. They'll be more patient and you'll feel less alone.

Give yourself time

For some, chemo brain fades after treatment. For others, it lingers. Be kind to yourself as your brain heals. You're not lazy or broken. You're healing.

The Emotional Impact of Chemo Brain

Losing your sharpness can feel like losing a part of who you were. For many of us, it's not just an inconvenience. It's a blow to our confidence. It's frustrating when your brain doesn't feel like it belongs to you anymore. It's exhausting to keep pretending you're fine when inside, you're mourning the old version of you. The one who could juggle a million things and still remember the grocery list.

Chemo brain can lead to feelings of:
* Embarrassment during conversations
* Shame when tasks take longer than they should
* Anxiety over forgetting something important
* Grief for the "you" that cancer took
* Depression, especially when you feel isolated or misunderstood

But let me remind you, you are not dumb. You're not broken. You are navigating life with a brain that's been through trauma. And it's still doing its very best.

Your intelligence hasn't left you. It's just had to reroute.

Be patient and kind to that version of yourself who's still learning how to function in a world that expects speed, clarity, and constant memory. You've been through something huge, and you're still here. You're still capable of showing up in beautiful, meaningful ways.

Brain Exercises to Help You Feel Sharper

Think of your brain like a muscle. It might be tired or slower than it used to be, but that doesn't mean it can't regain strength over time. Little by little, gentle mental stimulation can help rebuild confidence, improve focus, and restore clarity. You don't need to "train" your brain like an Olympic athlete. Just keep it moving.

Read short articles or listen to audiobooks

Start small. A few pages of a book. A short podcast. Even following a recipe step-by-step counts. It engages memory and attention.

Play word or number games

Try crossword puzzles, sudoku, word searches, or apps like Lumosity or Elevate. Just 5–10 minutes a day can help build mental agility.

Journal or write lists by hand

Writing activates different parts of the brain than typing. Try keeping a daily journal, gratitude list, or even doodling. It helps improve memory and reduces stress.

Practice recall

At the end of each day, try to list 3 things you did or saw. Over time, this builds memory recall without pressure.

Talk it out

Explain something you learned or read to someone else. Teaching or summarizing information helps reinforce what your brain is trying to hold onto.

Try guided meditation or mindfulness

Apps like Insight Timer or Calm offer short guided meditations. Focused breathing can improve clarity and reduce brain fog.

Learn something new (slowly)

Take a gentle online class, learn a new word daily, or try a new hobby. Just remember: it's okay if it doesn't stick right away. It's the trying that matters.

What Good Can Come From This?

It might seem laughable to suggest there's a silver lining in cancer treatment. And let me be clear, I'm not here to slap a sunshine sticker on top of something as brutal and soul-splitting as breast cancer. The pain and fear are real. The emotional fallout is absolutely real. But sometimes while walking through hell, in the ashes and silence, you stumble across something good. Something unexpected that wasn't even visible until everything else had been stripped away.

For some people, it's a deeper empathy. For others, it's learning how to say no, or how to finally say yes. It might be discovering your own strength. It might be a friendship that deepens in a way it never could have before. Sometimes it's learning how to slow down. How to listen. How to let people love you without feeling guilty.

And for me?

Well, my silver lining didn't look like a silver lining at first. It took me years to finally see it.

My then-husband would take me to chemo, hold my hand through the appointments, kiss my forehead, and play the part of the loving, supportive husband like he was auditioning for a Hallmark movie. Then he'd take me home, tuck me into bed, and walk out the door. Not to run errands. Not to clear his head. But to meet up with one of the many other women in his orbit.

No, that wasn't the silver lining. That was the shovel. The one that unearthed the truth I had been too exhausted to face: he didn't love me at my worst, which meant he sure as hell didn't deserve me at my healed, whole, rising-from-the-ashes best.

Cancer stripped me down to nothing. But in that emptiness, I found clarity. I left him. And for the first time in years, I stood on my own: wobbly and unsure, but standing all the same.

I spent the next nine years rebuilding. I got to really know and like the woman who had survived it all. I learned how to love her. I figured out what brought me peace, what made me laugh, and who I could trust with the softest parts of me. I learned how to be alone without being lonely. How to love without losing myself.

And wouldn't you know it, somewhere in the middle of all that self-discovery, life had something waiting for me.

Turns out, I'd almost crossed paths with my now-husband more times than either of us can count. We were part of the same biker group. We had the same close friends. We went to the same parties, probably danced to the same music in the same smoky bars, but somehow, we never met. Not until the timing was right. Not until we were both ready. After I had survived the storm, put myself back together, and learned exactly who I was again.

And when I met him, I knew. This man is my calm. My safe space and solid ground under my feet. He has never needed me to be anything other than exactly who I am. He doesn't disappear when things get hard. He grabs my hand and says, "Let's walk through this together." And I believe him, because he shows me. Every damn day.

And when I hit those moments where the emotions run too deep or the grief sneaks back in, he's not too proud to pick up the phone and call my best friend or my daughter and say, "She needs you." He knows when he's in over his head. That's real love. It's not just showing up when it's easy, it's knowing when to bring in backup, too.

So yeah, cancer took a lot from me. But it cleared away the brush and showed me the right path.

It made space for something better and introduced me to the strongest version of myself I've ever known, and somehow led me straight to the man who was always meant to walk beside me.

That's my silver lining. And I never would've found it if I hadn't made it through the fire.

💬 Quotes from Survivors

"I tried to do anything that needed real attention first thing in the day, not later when I was tired. And I simply did not even try on days one to two of weekly chemo. Days three through six were better for thinking."

—Julia, breast cancer survivor, on managing cognitive challenges during chemotherapy

"You can be sad. You can go there. But you can't stay there. Try to set your intention to get through the day and be as present as you can be."
—Heather Jose, cancer survivor, offering advice on emotional resilience during treatment

🖌 Chapter Highlights

- Side effects of treatment are more than physical. They affect your identity, your emotions, and your daily life.

- Hair loss can be one of the most emotional parts of chemotherapy, but options like cold capping may help some retain control.

- Taste changes, weight gain, bone pain, and "chemo brain" are common but also very personal experiences, and they deserve to be acknowledged and treated seriously.

- There are tools that can help manage side effects, from practical tips to emotional coping strategies. You're not expected to go through this alone or in silence.

- Tracking symptoms, asking questions, and adjusting treatment if needed are all part of advocating for your health.

🩶 Key Takeaway

This chapter is about reclaiming power in the face of what feels uncontrollable. It's about honoring every ache, every change, and every moment of "I don't recognize myself" with compassion instead of shame. You are enduring, and that matters.

"Every day you should do something kind for your body."
—Sheryl Crow; focused on environmental risk factors and screening access

8
Beyond the Basics:
Hormone, Targeted, & Immunotherapies

Not every treatment ends with chemo and radiation. For many of us, there's more—therapies that don't always get talked about in the same way but carry just as much weight. Hormone therapy, targeted therapy, and immunotherapy aren't always as visible, but they're powerful tools that continue working behind the scenes long after the last infusion or final surgery. They're used to block hormone signals, interrupt cancer cell growth, or help the immune system recognize and fight what doesn't belong.

And while these therapies can be life-saving, they also come with their own physical and emotional tolls. They don't always hit you all at once like chemo might, but their effects can be long, slow, and quietly brutal. For some, the hardest part isn't when the hair falls out or the radiation burns appear—it's when treatment keeps going and everyone assumes you're already "done."

Let's take a deeper look at these next steps.

Hormone (Endocrine) Therapy

"Tamoxifen gave me hot flashes, insomnia, and mood swings that made me feel like a stranger to myself. My family didn't know what to do with me." — Alicia M., on hormonal shifts and emotional regulation

"I didn't expect the fatigue to be that bad. I was done with chemo and thought things would get easier. But this was a different kind of tired. Like my bones were tired." — Renee T., on post-treatment exhaustion

I didn't complete hormone therapy, but I did start it. My doctor prescribed Tamoxifen and wanted me to take it for five years. I didn't make it six weeks.

To say my mood swings were out of control would be an understatement. They were disorienting. I knew I was reacting to things in ways that didn't make sense, even as it was happening. I knew, logically, that I was being unreasonable, but there didn't seem to be an off switch. At times, there was this overwhelming, volcanic rage bubbling up inside of me, and I had no idea where it was coming from. I remember standing in my kitchen, heart racing, hands trembling, absolutely filled with fury, and I didn't even know why. It scared me so badly that I stopped taking Tamoxifen right then and there.

Looking back now, I wonder how much of that spiral was caused by the medication, and how much was just the emotional wreckage of everything I hadn't yet dealt with. The trauma of cancer. The cracks in my marriage. The sheer emotional exhaustion I'd been carrying like an overloaded backpack. I hadn't faced any of it in a healthy way. I just kept going. Surviving. Kept pretending I was fine.

I remember once, being so angry at my husband, not just because he was cheating on me, but because one of the women he was cheating with actually showed up at my workplace. She came there to "confirm" what he had apparently told her: that he and I had agreed on an open relationship. Which, let me be very clear, we *absolutely had not*. That little gem was entirely his fiction. So when one of his friends, someone I thought would be neutral, stepped in to actually defend him? I snapped. I lost it. I slapped the friend, right there in the middle of everything.

I'm not proud of it. That's not who I am. I make jokes on Facebook about "Throat Chop Thursday," but it's just that. A joke. But I was so far past my limit that I didn't even recognize myself anymore. That moment felt like the explosion of everything I'd been bottling up: grief, rage, betrayal, confusion, hormones, trauma.

All of it was twisted together into one tangled, hot mess.

Yes, there were valid reasons to be upset in my marriage. But this chapter isn't really about that. It's about the *layers* of pain and confusion that breast cancer treatment can bring. It's about how hormone therapy, while often overshadowed by surgery, chemo, and radiation, can be just as defining.

Although I didn't stay on Tamoxifen and never received targeted or immunotherapy, I've spoken to so many women who have. And while these treatments can be life-saving, that doesn't mean they're easy. Far from it.

Some people tolerate them just fine, while others describe side effects that feel like they're slowly being unraveled. It's not the visible trauma of surgery, or the harsh, in-your-face toll of chemo. It's something more subtle. It is the slow erosion of energy, patience, memory, and of anything still feeling like your old self.

Take Sarah, for example. She was 42 when she was diagnosed with Stage 1, hormone receptor–positive breast cancer. After her surgery and radiation, her oncologist recommended five years of Tamoxifen. At first, she felt lucky. No chemo. No infusion center. Just one pill a day. It sounded manageable, like maybe she'd dodged the worst of it.

But the reality turned out to be more complicated than she had anticipated.

The hot flashes jolted her awake at night. Her joints started to ache like she'd aged 30 years overnight. Her moods shifted without warning. Her memory felt fuzzy, like walking into a room and forgetting why she was there, over and over again. Slowly, she found herself wondering if the pills meant to protect her were also stealing tiny pieces of her joy.

Still, she stuck with it. She worked closely with her doctor and eventually switched to an aromatase inhibitor. She began walking every morning to ease the stiffness and joined a support group for women on long-term hormone therapy.

"Some days," she told me, "I just wanted to be done. But then I'd remind myself that this little pill is part of what's keeping me here. And that helped."

This chapter isn't here to tell you what to do. It's not here to shame you if you stop or scare you into continuing. It's here to help you *understand*. To remind you that whatever you're feeling is valid. And that it's okay to ask questions. It's okay to talk to your doctor about side effects, and to advocate for changes if something isn't working.

Hormone therapy might be part of your path. It might not. Either way, you deserve full, honest conversations about what it means, physically, mentally, and emotionally.

Because knowledge is power. And you deserve to feel empowered every step of the way.

Questions to Ask:

- Is my tumor hormone receptor–positive?

- Which medication is right for my stage of life?

- How long will I need to take it (5, 7, or 10 years)?

- Will I need regular bone scans (DEXA)?

- What can I do to manage side effects?

Targeted Therapy

Targeted therapy focuses on the unique features of cancer cells rather than attacking all fast-growing cells like chemotherapy does. These drugs are designed to **"target" specific proteins or genes** that help cancer grow or spread. In HER2-positive breast cancer, for example, the drug **Herceptin (trastuzumab)** attaches to the HER2 receptors on cancer cells, blocking their growth and marking them for destruction by the immune system.

"I had HER2-positive cancer, so I took Herceptin. I thought it would be easier than chemo, but it came with its own baggage: headaches, chills, and just feeling 'off' most of the time." — Jillian B., on the hidden cost of targeted therapy

"I didn't realize I'd need heart scans for years after. Herceptin helped save me, but I still hold my breath every time I go in for a MUGA." — Melissa F., on the emotional toll of long-term monitoring
Targeted therapy is a more personalized approach. It's designed to go after specific proteins, like HER2, or genetic mutations that help cancer

112

grow. These drugs are like snipers because they look for the weak spot in the cancer's armor and go after it.

And while that precision sounds promising, these therapies can come with their own set of challenges.

Some women report feeling constantly fatigued, not in the way chemo knocks you down, but more like a slow leak. A consistent drain of energy that sneaks up on you. Diarrhea can be common, which may feel inconvenient at best and completely debilitating at worst. And because certain targeted therapies can stress the heart, regular scans like MUGA (a heart function test using a special camera) or echos become part of your new normal.

Still, there's hope in the specificity. Many people find encouragement in knowing that their treatment is based on their cancer's unique traits, not just a one-size-fits-all plan. That knowledge alone can be reassuring and empowering. Here, you're not just being treated. You're being understood.

Questions to Ask:

- Does my cancer have HER2 over expression or other targetable markers?

- Will I need heart scans (MUGA or echo) during treatment?

- What symptoms should I report immediately?

- How does this therapy fit into my overall treatment plan?

Immunotherapy

Note: While no contributors in this book shared their personal experience with immunotherapy, that absence is telling. This is a newer therapy, and many people are still navigating its uncertainties or haven't yet had access. If you're feeling unsure or alone in this part of your treatment, you're not alone in that feeling.

Immunotherapy is one of the newer cancer therapies, especially for breast cancer, and it's showing promising results, particularly for triple-negative types with PD-L1 expression. It works by boosting your immune system so it can better recognize and destroy cancer cells. It has the potential to be powerful and life-changing.

But ramping up your immune system also means it can become overzealous. Sometimes, it doesn't stop at attacking cancer cells. It can get confused and start targeting your healthy tissues, which is where autoimmune-type symptoms come in.

For some, this looks like persistent fatigue, rash, inflammation, or unexpected changes to the thyroid. It can also affect your joints, lungs, or digestive system. You may feel flu-like. Or just "off" in ways that are hard to explain. These symptoms are called immune-related adverse events, and they can be tricky because they don't always show up right away. Sometimes they creep in weeks or even months after treatment begins.

What makes immunotherapy different is its unpredictability. It's not always obvious when side effects will appear or how severe they'll be. But when it works, it can extend lives and offer new hope to people who previously had limited options. And that's no small thing.

It's okay to be both hopeful and cautious. To feel a combination of brave and scared.

Questions to Ask:

- Am I eligible for immunotherapy or any clinical trials?

- What are the risks and benefits for my cancer subtype?

- Will this be used alone or with chemo?

Navigating the Journey Ahead

If you're stepping into hormone therapy, targeted therapy, or immunotherapy, it's possible you're already worn down from whatever treatments that came before. Maybe you're exhausted, or numb, and you're just trying to get through one more step in a journey that feels like it's never-ending.

These therapies are powerful and are often the unsung heroes working in the background long after the surgery scars have healed and the last drop of chemo has been infused. But their strength doesn't always make you feel like the warrior you are. Sometimes, it feels like a trade-off. Your comfort, your emotions, your energy, for a few more guarded steps into the future.

And that's a hard bargain to live with every day.

The emotional tolls that these therapies take on a person aren't discussed enough. The mood swings that come out of nowhere. The mental fog that settles in. The slow, quiet questioning of who you are now, and asking, "Is it worth it?" You may look "done" with treatment to everyone else, but inside, it can feel like the hardest part is just beginning.

Please hear this: what you're feeling is real. It's normal and your feelings are valid. You should ask for help when you need it. Get coffee and vent to a friend, talk to your doctor, or find a therapist who understands your situation. Connect with others who've walked this path, either in person or online. You don't have to carry this part of the journey on your own.

Whether you complete the full course of treatment or not, you are still fighting. You're still healing. And you are always worthy of compassion and care, especially from yourself.

There is no perfect way through this. Only your way. And whatever that looks like, it's enough. YOU are enough. Keep going.

✔ Chapter Highlights

- Hormone therapy, like Tamoxifen or aromatase inhibitors, can cause significant side effects but remains a key long-term treatment for hormone receptor–positive cancers.

- Targeted therapy attacks specific cancer traits, like HER2 over expression, and may require ongoing heart monitoring and side effect management.

- Immunotherapy works by boosting your immune system to fight cancer but can trigger autoimmune-like side effects that may appear unexpectedly.

- Each therapy comes with its own emotional and physical toll. Feeling overwhelmed doesn't mean you're weak.

- These therapies often extend far beyond visible treatment and deserve just as much support, attention, and validation.

🩶 Key Takeaway

This chapter is about the silent battles that follow the big ones. The pills, infusions, and invisible side effects can leave you feeling forgotten, but you're still fighting, still healing, and still deserving of care, every step of the way.

"There's a hope that's waiting for you in the dark.
You should know you're beautiful just the way you are.
And you don't have to change a thing,
the world could change its heart.
No scars to your beautiful,
we're stars and we're beautiful."
—Alessia Cara, Scars to Your Beautiful

9

The Heart of Healing

There's a part of cancer no one really talks about. It's not as visible as the scars or as easy to name as the side effects printed on a prescription bottle. We cover the surgeries, the appointments, the medications. We talk about the hair loss, the exhaustion, the waiting rooms and insurance claims. But we rarely talk about the emotional wreckage; the kind that doesn't show up on a scan.

It's not just the patient who suffers. The whole family feels it. The silence between couples when they don't know what to say. The fog that settles over the household like a thick, heavy blanket. The way everything might look normal on the outside, while inside, things are slowly breaking apart.

When my mom offered to come down from Michigan to help, I told her no. I said we had it handled. But the truth is, I had no idea how to let people help me. I was stuck in performance mode, trying so hard to be strong and composed that I didn't even notice I was quietly crumbling.

My husband and I were both military veterans, trained to be tough. Trained to adapt and overcome. Trained to never complain. But no amount of military discipline prepares you for emotional landmines. What we didn't know how to talk about was our fear. We didn't know how to talk about grief or helplessness. So, we just didn't. We slowly escaped into our own silences, our own distractions.

For me, that escape became alcohol.

At first, it was innocent enough. A drink here and there, just to take the edge off the anxiety and the noise in my head. But slowly, that soft buzz became my emotional security blanket. I drank to quiet the silence. I drank to soften the loneliness. I drank to survive the grief of losing parts of myself I wasn't ready to let go of: my body, my womanhood, my sense of normalcy. Not because I was an alcoholic, but because I was drowning.

His escape looked different. His came in the form of women: flirting, affairs, secret messages, and late-night disappearances. In a world that had spun completely out of his control, I think seeking comfort elsewhere made him feel powerful again. Or maybe just distracted. Either way, it broke something between us that couldn't be repaired.

I finally broke down halfway through radiation. I couldn't carry the pressure inside anymore. I checked myself into rehab, fully convinced that I had a drinking problem. But what I found there wasn't only detox, it was clarity. I met a therapist who looked me in the eye and told me the truth I hadn't been able to say out loud. She said I didn't have to be strong all the time. She assured me that I was allowed to fall apart. And for the first time in a long, long time, I exhaled. I let the armor crack, and I spoke the things I'd been stuffing down for months.

When I left rehab, I also left my marriage.

I walked away from the version of myself who thought she had to be strong for everyone around her. I walked away from the woman who made excuses for a man who betrayed her while she was at her most vulnerable. I walked away from the lie that healing could happen in the middle of a toxic storm.

I'm telling you this not because I want sympathy. And not because I think everyone's story looks like mine. I'm telling you because I want to catch you before you hit your own breaking point. Before your coping mechanism, whatever it might be, becomes your crisis.

You don't owe anyone your strength, and vulnerability is not weakness. It's how healing begins.

You're allowed to say, "I'm not okay," or "This is too much." You are allowed to feel everything, even the things that make other people uncomfortable.

Because let's be honest, this entire experience is exhausting. Cancer treatment isn't only a physical battle; it's a mental marathon. It demands more from you than you ever expected to give. You walk into a process that makes you feel worse before it makes you better, and you do it willingly. That takes guts. That takes grit. That takes *everything*.

Even when you're surrounded by love. Even when people show up for you. Even then, it's hard.

✒ Corinna B., Diagnosed at 44

I was 44 when the word "cancer" entered my world like a wrecking ball. Stage 1, HER2-positive. I'd already been worn thin with the fatigue, night sweats, constant stress that clung to me like a second skin. And then came treatment.

Chemo was six rounds of hell. The nausea wasn't just occasional, it lived with me. Some days the smell of food would turn my stomach; brushing my teeth made me gag. My bones ached deep at night, like they were splintering from the inside. My period, which had been gone, came crashing back during infusions. I bled through my clothes in public. I was embarrassed. Angry. No one told me to expect that.

The steroids made everything worse. I felt wired and restless, like my body couldn't figure out how to shut down. I'd lie in bed wide awake, buzzing with anxiety, staring at the ceiling while my heart raced. My mind spiraled, and sleep slipped further out of reach.

And then there was the hair. Long, thick, beautiful hair that fell out in clumps, and my scalp burned with a tenderness I hadn't expected. I held the razor in my hand and cried in front of the mirror. It felt like I was shaving off the last piece of myself that looked like me. And no one around me really seemed to understand just how much that moment broke my heart.

I told my husband, "I'm not okay." I said the words out loud, but even I didn't know how to explain what I meant. I felt invisible. Like I was screaming underwater and no one could hear me.

But something changed when I finally reached out for help. I started therapy. I got massages. I turned to meditation, not because it fixed everything, but because it gave me moments of stillness. Little by little, I found my way back to myself.

It was a long process, and I didn't just return to who I was before. I became someone stronger. More open. I don't take joy for granted now. I find it in the quietest corners, sunlight on my face, a long exhale, a

119

random moment of laughter that bubbles up and reminds me I'm still here.

Cancer stripped away so much, but in its place, I found depth and clarity. I found myself asking for help, saying what I needed, and refusing to apologize for it. Healing didn't come all at once, it came in layers. And with every layer, I grew into someone I actually like.

I'm not who I used to be. I'm someone braver.

✐ Amy M., Survivor of 18 Years

When I first heard the words "you have breast cancer," I didn't cry. I didn't crumble. I got mad.

Not just a little irritated. I was furious in that deep, bone-hot way where your whole body buzzes with adrenaline and disbelief. I had plans: races to run, vacations on the calendar, memories to make. And now I had to cancel everything because cancer had barged in, uninvited and unapologetic. There was no warning. It felt like someone slammed the brakes on my life, and all I could do was brace for impact.

I found the lump myself. It was small, but it didn't feel right. The diagnosis came quickly: Stage 1, but Grade 3. The most aggressive kind. I wasn't afraid, not yet. I didn't even cry at first. My emotions hadn't caught up with my reality. I was too busy shifting into gear, too focused on fighting. I think I treated it like a to-do list. Appointments. Treatments. Get it done. Keep moving.

But the feelings came later, in waves. Usually when it was quiet.

In the infusion room, the lights were always too bright and the air too cold, that sterile chill that seems to settle in your bones. The Red Devil, a nickname for one of the chemo drugs, was as brutal as it sounds. Bright, angry red in the IV bag. You could taste the chemicals in the back of your throat before they even finished dripping. Metallic. Sharp. Wrong. Later, your pee would turn red too, a haunting reminder of what had just been pumped into your veins. Poison, with the intention to save.

I sat in that chair four times. Four rounds of the strongest treatments they could give me. I remember watching the faces around me, week after week, and then realizing that some of those faces weren't coming back. That's when the anger shifted. It turned into something heavier. Sadder. Guiltier.

I kept running during chemo. Literally. Running races. Until the day my adductor muscle tore away from the bone. Even then, once it healed, I got back out there. I wasn't going to let cancer take that from me too.

I wore a scarf on my head instead of a wig. I couldn't stand the itch of synthetic hair. The scarf was soft, comforting, even when it drew stares. My students were curious. One of them asked if he could touch my head. I let him. His small hand felt warm and careful.

I spoke in front of 30,000 people at Detroit's Race for the Cure. I was more nervous standing on that stage than I ever was sitting in a chemo chair. But I did it. And for eleven years, I won that race. Every single time. That was my way of taking control back. My way of telling cancer it didn't get to define me.

My family and friends showed up the best they could, but sometimes we all pretended things were fine. I think we needed that. Sometimes the pretending was the only thing keeping us steady.

People say what doesn't kill you makes you stronger. And I guess it did. But I still carry all of it: the rage, the memories, the faces that never made it out of those chairs. It's all tucked in with me, somewhere quiet. Somewhere sacred.

Why Asking for Help Feels So Hard

There's this persistent myth floating around that therapy is only for people who are falling apart. Like it's some last resort you turn to when everything has come crashing down and you're clinging to the edge of rock bottom. But let me be clear, therapy isn't just for those on the verge. It's for anyone who wants more than just survival. It's for the ones who want to heal. Who want to understand. Who want to feel whole again, even if they don't quite know what that looks like yet.

You don't need to be in crisis to ask for help. Your life doesn't need to be in flames before you reach out and say, "Hey, I could use someone to talk to." That mindset kept me stuck for a long time.

It took me 17 years to write this book. Not because I didn't have the words, but because I never took the time to sit with the pain long enough to untangle it. I didn't seek help for the trauma. I didn't talk it through. I tried to outrun it. Tried to outwork it. I kept myself busy and buried until the healing I desperately needed was delayed by almost two decades. I had to figure things out on my own. I had to wrestle with questions like "Why me?" and "Did I do something to deserve this?" And I had to answer those questions without anyone holding space for me while I cried or screamed or simply sat in the silence.

And I know I'm not the only one.

One woman I spoke to, living with stage 4 breast cancer, shared something with me that I'll never forget. Her young son had stopped sleeping through the night. He was tired, withdrawn, struggling in school. When the school counselor gently asked him why, he whispered, "Because I'm afraid my mommy's going to die while I'm asleep."

That is just heartbreaking and screams, *this family needs support.*

Therapy isn't just for patients. It's not just for those with scars and diagnoses and medical charts a mile long. It's for the spouses who are holding their breath and trying to be brave. It's for the kids who don't know how to put fear into words. It's for the best friends, the adult daughters, the parents, the partners, the caregivers. Anyone walking this path deserves a safe space to unpack it all.

Cancer doesn't just grow in a body. It grows in the cracks of a family. In the unanswered questions. In the whispered fears and the unsaid grief. Therapy helps clear some of that debris. It helps you find your way back to yourself.

So if you've been wondering whether it's worth trying, let me say this with every bit of love and honesty I have: yes. Yes, it is. Whether you need help untangling the past, coping with the present, or imagining a future that feels safe again, therapy can hold that space. Please ask for help, not because you're falling apart, but because you're worth the effort it takes to put yourself back together.

When Faith Is the Therapy

Not everyone processes their trauma through therapy. And that's okay too.

My friend Joyce never stepped foot in a therapist's office. Not once. She didn't feel the need. For her, peace came from her faith, her family, and the unshakable support of her community. While some of us had to dig deep, unravel the knots, and crawl our way through the healing process, Joyce found her footing in a different way.

She had a husband who showed up, not just at appointments, but in the quiet moments in between. She had kids who saw her pain and helped without being asked. She had coworkers who dropped off gift baskets and casseroles, and church members who left envelopes of cash tucked into her mailbox, often at the exact moment she needed to book a hotel or fill up the gas tank for treatment. She didn't have peace because it was easy. She had peace because she trusted her people, her faith, her God, and she let them carry her when she couldn't carry herself.

Joyce's story isn't mine. But that's the beauty of it. Healing doesn't look the same for all of us.

Some of us need to talk until the words stop hurting. Some need to move, to write, to pray, to sit in silence. Some of us need to scream into pillows or cry on long drives with the music way too loud. And some, like Joyce, just need the steady beat of a life already rooted in something solid.

There is no one right way to heal.

If your peace comes from prayer, lean into it. If writing helps clear your mind, don't stop journaling. If talking is how you work things out, find someone to listen, whether it's a therapist, a friend, or someone who simply *gets it*. If you need solitude, claim it. If you need people, gather them.

The goal isn't to follow a perfect map. The goal is to find peace. However you find it.

And however long it takes.

Helping the Ones Around You

Children pick up on more than we give them credit for. Even when we think we're shielding them, whispering in the next room, keeping the tears behind closed doors, they feel it. They feel the shifts in our energy, the weight of our silence, the undercurrent of fear. And often, they don't have the words to name what they're sensing. That's where therapy can be a lifeline. Not because something is "wrong" with them, but because it gives them space to explore and express the things they don't know how to ask out loud.

There are different forms of therapy for different ages and stages. Play therapy is especially helpful for little ones, offering them a safe outlet through toys, drawing, and imagination. It's about helping them process what's going on in a way their young minds can understand. For older kids and teens, school counselors and child psychologists can offer support in more traditional ways, helping them navigate the emotional rollercoaster they might be quietly riding. And sometimes, just having an adult outside of the family to talk to can make all the difference.

If you have kids in your life, don't be afraid to reach out and see what resources are available in your area. Many schools have support systems in place, and community centers or hospitals often have low-cost or sliding-scale therapy options for families affected by cancer.

And let's not forget the caregivers.

Whether it's a spouse, a partner, a parent, a sibling, or a best friend, cancer affects them too. Watching someone you love go through treatment, feeling helpless to ease their pain, walking that tightrope between showing strength and quietly falling apart—that's its own kind of trauma. Caregivers carry so much of the emotional weight behind the scenes, often without being asked, often without complaint. But that doesn't mean they're not struggling.

Therapy gives caregivers a space to breathe. To unravel. To cry or rage or admit they're scared, too. It gives them permission to talk about the guilt they feel when they need a break or the impossible questions they ask themselves at night, like *why them and not me?* It gives them a way to process their grief and fear without feeling like they're adding to yours.

Because when it comes right down to it, healing isn't just for the person in the hospital gown. It's for everyone in the blast radius.

We all deserve space to talk. To feel. To heal.

Emotional Whiplash: Naming the Feelings

You might feel everything. You might feel nothing. That's normal. Emotions after a diagnosis come in waves:

- Shock & Numbness: Like your brain pulled the emergency brake.

- Fear: A pit in your stomach that never quite goes away.

- Anger: At doctors, your body, God, the world.

- Sadness & Grief: Mourning your old self, your energy, your plans.

- Guilt: For not catching it sooner, for being a burden.

- Loneliness: Even in a crowded room, you feel alone.

- Frustration & Powerlessness: When control slips through your fingers.

- Hope & Resilience: When, somehow, you still keep going.

- Acceptance: When the noise quiets and you start to breathe again.

These feelings don't follow a script. They circle back. They crash unexpectedly. They teach you things you never asked to learn. But every one of them is survivable.

If Therapy Feels Too Big

If the idea of therapy feels overwhelming, like one more thing on an already impossible list, you're not alone. Healing doesn't have to start with a deep, tear-filled session in a stranger's office. You don't have to sit on a couch and bare your soul if that doesn't feel right yet.

Start smaller.

Maybe that means scribbling thoughts into a journal, just to get them out of your head. Maybe it's joining a Facebook group where people just *get it* without you needing to explain. Maybe it's taking five quiet minutes to breathe deeply or stretch your body. Talk to a chaplain. Try a podcast on mindfulness. Ask your cancer center if they offer counseling or support groups. There are more options out there than you might realize. And if none of them feel like the right fit yet, that's okay too.

You're allowed to ease into your healing. You're allowed to take your time. You've already survived the hardest parts. There's no deadline on what comes next.

Trauma and Triggers: When Little Things Feel Big

It might happen when you least expect it. The beeping of a hospital monitor on a TV show. The sharp smell of antiseptic. The feel of those flimsy gowns. Suddenly, your body tenses, your breath catches, and your heart starts racing because in that split second, you're there again. Back in the chemo chair. Back in the scan room. Back in the moment your life changed.

This is trauma.

Your nervous system remembers what you've been through, even if your mind tries to move on. This is a form of PTSD that many survivors experience, but rarely talk about.

Erin told me, "To this day, the sound of hospital beeping makes my heart race. I had a panic attack during my daughter's check-up because the monitor sounded exactly like the chemo pump. I thought I was losing it. Turns out, it's PTSD. Real, ugly, inconvenient PTSD."

You may find yourself panicking in a setting that seems completely benign to everyone else. Or avoiding certain buildings. Or sobbing during a routine doctor visit without even knowing why. All of it is normal. All of it makes sense.

Denise described the emotional crash that came after treatment. "Everyone thinks you're fine once the treatment ends. But that's when it hit me the hardest. I couldn't stop crying. Couldn't sleep. I jumped at every phone call, every twinge in my body. I was exhausted and terrified, and no one seemed to understand why."

Trauma doesn't always scream. Sometimes it whispers. Sometimes it hides in hyper-vigilance: the constant scanning of your body for what might go wrong next. The fear that never fully lets go.

Bri told me, "I thought surviving would be this huge relief. But instead, I became obsessed with every ache, every mole, every new freckle. I kept waiting for the other shoe to drop. I still do."

The good news is that your brain and body can heal. Tools like grounding exercises, breath work, movement, art, EMDR, and trauma-informed therapy can help you process those trapped experiences. And not all therapy looks the same; there are many different types. It's important to find what works for you. Whether that means talking it through, moving it through your body, writing it down, or simply naming it aloud.

What matters most is giving yourself grace, patience, and the space to heal in your own time. There is no timeline. There is no race.

Post-Traumatic Growth

There's a phrase I came across a few years after treatment that stuck with me: *post-traumatic growth*.

It doesn't mean you're grateful that the cancer happened. It doesn't mean you'd ever want to relive it. But it *does* mean you've come out the other side changed; not just in body, but in soul.

Maybe now you love deeper. Laugh louder. Set firmer boundaries. Forgive yourself quicker. Maybe now you savor quiet moments, or finally say the things you've been holding in for years. Maybe now, you understand your worth in a way you never did before.

Growth doesn't erase the scars. It doesn't undo the pain. But sometimes something beautiful blooms right in the middle of the wreckage. A version of you that's softer, stronger, wiser. Not in spite of what you've been through, but because you've survived it.

Nicole told me, "Before cancer, I never said no. I bent myself in half trying to make everyone else comfortable. But now I say no without guilt. Cancer taught me that my peace matters."

Jasmine shared something similar. "I used to race through life like I was being chased. Now, I sit on the porch with my tea and just *breathe*. Cancer didn't make me grateful, but it did make me still. I don't want to miss things anymore."

And Lena's words stayed with me for days. "I didn't recognize myself after treatment; not just physically, but emotionally. But over time, I realized I'd been wearing a mask for years. Cancer ripped it off. What's left is more *me* than I've ever been."

Chapter Highlights

- Cancer causes emotional trauma that can affect the patient and everyone close to them.

- Therapy is not weakness. It's a powerful tool for healing.

- Faith, community, and connection are equally valid paths to peace.

- Emotions after diagnosis are complex and constantly shifting.

- Children and caregivers need support too.

- You don't have to heal alone, and you don't have to heal in one particular way.

💜 **Key Takeaway**

You don't have to be strong all the time. Letting yourself feel, fall apart, and be seen is not failure. It's healing.

"You can't scare me. I've been through cancer."
— Hoda Kotb; advocated for positive mindset; supported awareness campaigns

10
Journaling, Mindfulness, & Meaning

Not all healing happens in hospitals or sick beds. Some of it happens in silence, when the world finally slows down and you're left alone with your thoughts. It can happen in the early hours of the morning, in the parking lot before an appointment, or at night when everyone else is asleep and you finally let yourself breathe. This chapter is about that quiet, internal work that helps you find your footing again.

Journaling: Writing to Heal

Journaling was one of the first tools I reached for, years after treatment, but still very much in the midst of healing. Writing helped me untangle all the thoughts that had been trapped in my head for far too long. It gave me permission to feel without having to explain or perform. Whether you're writing to share your thoughts, or to just get them out of your head, it can be a great way to work through your thoughts and emotions.

If you don't know where to begin, just think about how you're feeling. Even if all you can write is, "I don't know what to say," that's okay. Some of the most powerful moments come from putting something on paper, on your computer, or even in a blog.

Writing helps you:

- Slow down your thoughts

- Notice patterns in your emotions

- Release the fear or sadness you've been holding

- Track your growth over time

You don't need to be a professional writer. You just need to be honest with yourself about how you're feeling.

131

Types of journaling that might help:

- Free writing: no editing, no filter, just write.

- Prompted journaling: Use questions from the workbook to guide you.

- Letters to yourself, or your body, or even to fear itself.

- Gratitude lists, because even small ones count.

- Reflection after appointments or hard conversations.

There's no wrong way to do this. The goal is expression, not perfection.

✎ Heather R., Diagnosed at 42

I was 42 when I went in for my very first mammogram. Just a routine screening. No symptoms. No concerns. I almost skipped it. Life was busy, and who really wants to schedule a boob squish between errands? But I went. The next day, I got the call: "We need you to come back." And just like that, I was launched into a world I wasn't ready for.

It started with a mix of "Oh crap" and "Okay… here we go." But what followed was a mental tilt-a-whirl. After the biopsy, after the official diagnosis of Invasive Ductal Carcinoma with areas of DCIS, ER+/PR+, Stage 2A, I was handed an emotional buffet of treatment paths and expected to choose wisely. I second-guessed everything. One minute I was sure. The next I was spiraling. It felt like my brain had a thousand browser tabs open, each one playing a different anxiety soundtrack.

Ultimately, I decided on a double mastectomy. No reconstruction. Flat. It wasn't a decision I made lightly. It was a thousand tiny decisions that finally led me to one big, freeing yes. Choosing to go flat felt like reclaiming my body. No more trying to meet someone else's idea of what I should look like. I'd been through enough. I didn't owe anyone breasts to feel whole.

Recovery was a roller coaster. I prepped my house like a nesting mama bear before surgery. I moved everything I could to "T-Rex height" so I wouldn't have to reach up: coffee mugs, snacks, phone charger, even my favorite fuzzy socks. The post-op fog was real, but so were the moments of absurd humor. My dogs lovingly tripped me, my son made me laugh until I cried, and I wore a "Shitty Titty" shirt to work just to get ahead of the awkward conversations.

Journaling became my lifeline. I'd pour out every swirling, jumbled thought of rage, relief, exhaustion, gratitude. At some point, those scribbles started turning into something bigger. A memoir, maybe. A roadmap for someone else who needed to hear, "You're not alone. You're not broken. You're still you."

Mindfulness: Coming Back to the Present

Mindfulness is a word that gets thrown around a lot, but what it really means is being present. Being aware of what's happening inside you and around you, without judgment.

When you're dealing with cancer, your brain spends a lot of time in the past (what just happened?) or the future (what if it comes back?). Mindfulness invites you to come back to now; the only place where healing happens.

It doesn't require silence, incense, or sitting cross-legged for an hour. It can be as simple as taking three deep breaths and noticing your feet on the floor. Taking a walk and feeling the cool breeze. Calling a friend and enjoying a laugh. Slow down to think about how your senses are being used in that moment.

Ways to practice mindfulness:

- Box Breathing: Inhale for 4, hold for 4, exhale for 4, hold for 4.

- Body Scans: Close your eyes and pay attention to each part of your body, without judgment.

- Five-Senses Grounding: Name 5 things you see, 4 you can touch, 3 you hear, 2 you smell, 1 you taste.

- Mindful walks: Feel the ground beneath your feet. Notice the colors around you.

- Mindful eating or showering: Slow down and actually experience the moment.

You don't need to "clear your mind." You just need to notice it. Mindfulness is about creating space between you and your emotions, so you can respond instead of react.

⊚ Meaning: When Life Doesn't Make Sense

There's almost always a moment in the cancer journey when the question finally surfaces: "Why?"
Why me? Why now? Why this?

Sometimes the silence that follows that question is deafening. There isn't always an answer that makes sense. Sometimes there's no answer at all. But every once in a while, if you give it time, if you let the dust settle and the chaos quiet, you start to see something clearer. Not a justification, and definitely not a silver bow tied neatly around your pain, but maybe... a thread. A connection. A reason that feels more like a quiet knowing than an explanation.

That's how it happened for me.

I've talked before about how cancer cleared the path for me to really *know* myself again, and eventually led me to the love I have now. But there was a deeper layer of meaning that took years to understand. Looking back, I truly believe God gave me cancer because I didn't have the courage to leave my toxic marriage on my own. We had two daughters. He didn't hit me or hurt me in any physical way. With him, it was all mind games. Twisting the truths and gaslighting. And so, like so many women, I convinced myself I had to stay. I told myself it wasn't "that bad." I convinced myself that our daughters needed a full, whole family to grow up in. But deep down, I knew it was breaking me. I knew he was manipulative and vindictive. I knew leaving would be messy. Painful. Scary. So I stayed.

Until cancer forced everything to the surface.

When the diagnosis came, there was no more room to ignore the truth. There was no more pretending we were okay. Cancer didn't just expose what was going on in my body; it exposed what was broken in my life.

134

And as strange as it may sound, I knew that if I was going to survive this disease, I couldn't keep living a lie. I couldn't stay in that marriage. I couldn't keep playing a role to make everyone else comfortable while I was dying inside.

Cancer didn't just save my life.
It gave me my life *back*.

Now, I want to be really clear about something. This isn't about romanticizing illness. I'm not suggesting that pain always has a purpose or that everyone will walk away from cancer with some magical revelation. Meaning is deeply personal. It doesn't come wrapped in a Hallmark card. It can take years to form, and even then, it might never arrive in a way that makes the pain feel "worth it."

But for some of us, meaning doesn't erase the suffering. It simply gives it a shape. A context. A whisper of, *this mattered*.

So if you're still stuck in the "why" of it all, that's okay. You don't have to rush to figure it out. And you don't have to assign meaning to your pain if it doesn't sit right with you. But if, someday, something shifts and you start to see a sliver of light in the rubble… let it in. Let it grow. Let it tell you something new about who you are and where you're going.

Even the worst storms sometimes clear a path we never knew we needed.

You might ask yourself:

- What has changed in me since my diagnosis?

- What am I no longer willing to tolerate?

- What relationships have become clearer?

- Have I found a new sense of purpose or strength?

- What do I want to do with the time I have now?

Some people find meaning in their faith. Others find it in helping others, creating art, or simply living more wholesomely. You don't need to have all the answers. You just need to keep asking the questions.

⚘ Healing in Your Own Way

You don't have to journal. You don't have to meditate. You don't have to assign meaning to your pain. These are all just suggestions to help you find your way through the complicated season you're experiencing. You may very well come up with your own way to cope with the feelings involved with your cancer diagnosis.

But if any of these things feel like they might help, I want you to know they're here for you. And that it's okay to take your time. Healing doesn't look the same for everyone.

You might write a little, cry a lot, sit quietly, scream into a pillow, or find peace on a park bench watching the birds. All of it counts if it just lets you breathe easier for a while.

Dana told me, "I started writing in a notebook just to keep track of appointments, but it turned into something else. Rage, grief, gratitude: it all ended up on the page. I didn't share it with anyone. But those pages caught every tear I didn't want to cry in front of my kids."

Selena made healing its own kind of music. "I made a playlist for every mood: sad, angry, brave, numb. Some days I just laid on the floor and let it play. Other days I danced like my life depended on it. Maybe it did."

And Jo reminded me that healing doesn't have to look like anything big. "I found this bench at the park where the same bluebird came every morning. I'd sit there with my coffee and cry. Then I'd laugh. Then I'd cry again. I didn't call it healing, but I think it was."

🖋 Chapter Highlights:

- Journaling makes room for honest reflection and emotional release.

- Mindfulness helps you return to the present moment and reduce fear.

- Meaning doesn't make cancer okay, but it can make life feel more purposeful.

- There's no one "right" or "wrong" way to heal. Your path is your own.

🩶 Key Takeaway

You may not have chosen this journey, but you still get to decide how you walk it. Journaling, mindfulness, and meaning are not solutions — they're companions. And they can help guide you back to yourself.

"I'm clear, and that's a big word to me."
-Christina Applegate; founded Right Action for Women for free MRIs; promoted genetic testing awareness.

11
Saying It Out Loud

It happened in the Target parking lot. I was sitting in my yellow Jeep when the phone rang. Just an ordinary afternoon. Nothing special. I wasn't braced for bad news. I wasn't holding anyone's hand or sitting in a sterile office. I wasn't prepared in any way.

And then, just like that, I had cancer.

The words didn't feel real at first. My ears started ringing before my brain could catch up. The doctor kept talking, but I only heard pieces. Fragments. Something about what it was and what the next steps would be. None of it landed. My mind had already floated somewhere else. Somewhere numb and out of reach.

I got off the phone and sat there. Just sat, looking at the steering wheel. The outside world didn't stop around me, but mine did, inside that car.

And then I called my husband. Then my mom. I told them the news, though I couldn't tell you what words I used. I didn't plan it. I didn't think it through. I just... said it. Like I was reading lines in a play.

The truth hadn't hit me yet. It was like my voice belonged to someone else. I hadn't even cried. Was I still breathing?

And after that, I went into Target.

I walked the aisles, dazed, putting things in my cart that I didn't need, half-aware of my body, my surroundings, the bright overhead lights that felt too sharp. I didn't tell anyone. I didn't fall apart or scream or crumble into a puddle.

I remained among strangers. Anonymous.

Because I didn't know what else to do.

Looking back, I still can't believe that's how I found out. That someone just called me. Dropped it into my lap like a forgotten appointment reminder. No warning. No sit-down with my husband beside me. No gentle explanation or kind voice in a quiet office. Just a cold, clinical sentence that changed my life.

And then I was expected to function. To tell people. To hold *their* hands through *my* news. To help *them* digest *my* crisis.

If you've just been diagnosed, you might feel like the world just cracked open to swallow you whole, while no one even noticed. You might not even know how to say the words out loud yet. Or maybe you already blurted them out in a moment of shock and now you're wondering if you did it wrong.

Let me tell you this: There's no easy way to say *"I have cancer."* No graceful script or magic formula.

There is only your truth, and the bravery it takes to speak it, even when your voice shakes.

My experience wasn't unique in its shock, but it was personal. And yet, I've heard others describe those first moments with the same dazed disbelief, as if the ground dropped out from under them while the rest of the world just kept spinning.

✎ **Melissa W**. received her diagnosis via MyChart at 8 p.m. on a Saturday night. The screen may have delivered the words, but it was the phone call from her doctor-friend that helped her breathe again. Even in the thick of shock, that voice reminded her she wasn't alone.

This chapter won't give you a cheat sheet, but it will give you permission to be honest and stay true to yourself during one of the scariest times of your life. This chapter is to tell you that it's okay to not know what to say. You can let others in anyway. We'll walk through the moments ahead. How to talk to loved ones, what to expect, and how to keep showing up even when your heart is still catching up with your words.

Let's Start With This: You Don't Owe Anyone a Performance

You don't have to be stoic or brave. You don't even need to use a calm voice if you're falling apart on the inside. It's perfectly normal to feel scared, unsure, or even numb when you say the words. This isn't a script for a tv show. This is your life.

Why It Matters to Tell People

There was a time, not that long ago, when breast cancer was spoken about in hushed tones, if at all. Women carried their diagnoses like secrets. They didn't talk about their breasts out loud and many felt breast cancer was some sort of punishment for imagined wrongs. They whispered about it in church parking lots or never said a word at all. Some suffered in silence and many died in it. And generations later, their daughters and granddaughters were left without answers, without knowing they were at risk too.

For some, it was shame. For others, fear. And for many, it was simply how they were taught: we don't talk about these things.

Even now, that silence lingers. Some of us instinctively go quiet, not wanting to worry our families, not knowing what to say, or feeling like we'll be judged for not being strong enough. We don't want to burden anyone. We don't want to be pitied. So we pull inward. We put on a smile and say, "I'm fine," even when we're falling apart inside.

But silence doesn't protect you. It does the opposite by isolating you at a time when you could use all the support you can get.

Telling someone you have cancer isn't about making them uncomfortable. It's about making yourself seen. It's about connection, clarity, and care.

When you speak the truth, out loud, you give people the chance to show up for you. And when you write down your diagnosis, your treatment plan, your experiences, you're doing more than tracking your journey. You're creating a record. A breadcrumb trail. Something your children, your siblings, or even your future self might one day need.

I can't tell you how many times I wished I could ask my mom more questions about her health. She had a hysterectomy years ago, but she never explained why. When I asked my dad, he didn't know either. And now she's gone, and so are those answers.

You deserve more. Your loved ones do too.

So speak. Even if it's hard. Even if your voice cracks. Even if all you can say at first is, "Something's wrong, and I'm scared."

Because when you open that door, even just a little, you create space for love to walk in. And that might be one of the most healing things of all.

✎ **Belinda** learned of her diagnosis by phone too. Afterward, she didn't launch into calls or gather her family. She just sat there and cried. Then, when she had gathered herself enough, she sent a single text to her children and grandson: "I'm trying to process everything. I'll call in a couple of days." She needed time. And that was okay. It was her way of catching her breath.

💬 How to Tell the People Closest to You

There's no one-size-fits-all way to say, "I have cancer." But there are ways to make the moment more bearable for you and for the people who love you.

You don't have to rehearse in front of a mirror like a monologue, and you don't need perfect timing or poetic words. What you do need is a little space, a little clarity, and the reminder that you are allowed to do this your way.

Here are a few gentle suggestions to help you prepare:

🕯 Choose the Right Setting

Tell them somewhere safe and quiet, where there's time to sit, cry, ask questions, or even sit in silence. Avoid breaking the news when someone is rushing to work or juggling distractions. If it has to be a phone call, make sure you are in a calm place first.

🗣 Start Simple and Honest

You don't have to spill everything at once. This isn't a press conference. Try something like:

"I've just gotten some news I need to share, and I'm still processing it myself. I've been diagnosed with breast cancer."

Then take a breath. Let the moment be what it is. If they cry, let them. If they ask questions that you're unsure about, you can say, "I don't know yet, but I'll tell you when I do." You are not required to carry their emotions too.

⊘ Offer a Role, Not a Script

Most people feel helpless after hearing news like this. They want to do something, but they don't know how. If you're comfortable, give them a role:

"Can you come with me to my next appointment?" "I might need help with meals in a couple weeks. Can I reach out?" "Right now, I just need you to sit with me."

This makes them feel useful. Connected. Included. It lets love have a job.

🙏 Expect a Range of Reactions

Some people will hug you and weep. Others will go quiet. Some will ask too many questions. A few might panic and blurt something ridiculous. (Trust me, I've heard some doozies.)

And some may pull away altogether; not out of malice, but fear. Cancer scares people, especially those who've lost someone. It brings up their own unhealed grief and uncertainty. If they need space, it's okay to let them have it, for now.

Later in this chapter, we'll talk more about those who distance themselves and how to hold space for that too.

But right now, just focus on the people who lean in. The ones who text back. Who say, "I don't know what to say, but I'm here." Those are your people.

🧰 When to Tell Your Employer

Telling your employer that you've been diagnosed with cancer can feel almost as daunting as telling your family. It's not just personal, it's professional. There are concerns about your job, your privacy, your income, and how people at work might treat you.

Let's take a breath and walk through this together.

🕐 Timing Is Yours

You don't have to tell your employer immediately, especially if you're still processing the news yourself. But if your treatment will impact your schedule, stamina, or ability to perform certain tasks, it's helpful to share sooner rather than later.

This gives you space to advocate for yourself and get the support you need.

🗣 What to Say

You don't owe them your full medical history. What you do need to share is enough to help them understand what's changing, and what accommodations you may need.

Here's a simple, professional approach:

"I want to let you know that I've recently been diagnosed with breast cancer. I'll be undergoing treatment in the coming weeks, which may affect my schedule and energy levels. I'm committed to continuing my work and would appreciate any flexibility we can build in as I navigate this."

From there, you can talk about specifics: time off for appointments, adjusted deadlines, temporary remote work, or reduced hours.

🧾 Know Your Rights

You are legally protected. Here are a few resources to explore:

- **FMLA (Family and Medical Leave Act):** Allows eligible employees to take up to 12 weeks of unpaid, job-protected leave.

- **Short-Term Disability Insurance:** If you have it through your employer, this can provide partial income during treatment.

- **ADA (Americans with Disabilities Act):** May entitle you to reasonable accommodations without penalty.

Don't be afraid to ask for a meeting with HR if you need help understanding your options. This isn't just about what you're entitled to; it's about building a work environment that supports your healing.

Be Gentle With Yourself

Some people find comfort in working. It gives a sense of normalcy. Others need time and space to rest, reset, and cope. There's no right or wrong way to approach work during this chapter. Just your way.

And whatever you choose, you're not letting anyone down.

Navigating Awkward Conversations (AKA: The Social Minefield of Cancer)

There's something about the word *cancer* that makes people glitch like a robot in a rainstorm. You say it, and suddenly their face freezes, their eyes dart around like they're searching for the emergency exit, and you can practically hear the Microsoft error sound playing inside their head. The air gets weird. Their voice gets weird. *Everything* gets weird.

And then they speak.

What follows is often a word salad of unsolicited advice, outdated clichés, or personal trauma they apparently couldn't wait to share. You might get the perky "You've got this!" or the spiritual "Everything happens for a reason." Some launch into their great-aunt's horror story, one that ends badly, by the way. And then others go full ghost. Like your diagnosis might somehow slip through the phone lines and infect their weekend plans.

It's disorienting. It's exhausting. And it's definitely not your job to soothe their emotional whiplash.

The thing is, cancer cracks people open in a way they weren't prepared for. It reminds them that life is fragile, that bodies fail, that control is an illusion. And for many, that fear gets projected right back onto you in the form of cringe-inducing comments or uncomfortable distance. Their awkwardness isn't a reflection of your worth, it's a reflection of their own inability to sit with discomfort.

Still… that doesn't make it any less frustrating.

🌀 Don't Make It Weird (But People Will Anyway)

Look, people mean well. They do. But when you have cancer, it's like you've become public property. Your diagnosis gives folks some imaginary permission slip to say whatever pops into their heads, and wow, do they run with it.

Let's break down some of the classics:

😳 The Unhelpful Optimist

- "You're so strong!"

- "Everything happens for a reason."

- "Just stay positive!"

Reality check: This isn't a yoga retreat. You're not manifesting your tumor away with vision boards and green juice. It's okay to be scared, pissed, tired, or numb. Responses like, "Thanks, I'm taking it one step at a time," work well. Or, if you're feeling feisty, try: "If positivity cured cancer, I'd be glowing like a damn unicorn by now."

🐾 The Over-sharer

- "My aunt had that! It spread to her brain…"

- "My friend's coworker's cousin died from that."

Boundaries, babe. This isn't open mic night for medical horror. A gentle "I'm trying to stay focused on my own treatment right now" can redirect the convo. Or just go full savage: "Wow. That's... a lot. I think I'm good on cancer death stories today, thanks."

The Vanisher

- Stops texting.

- Avoids eye contact at work.

- Disappears like you're cursed.

Oof. This one stings. But their disappearance usually says more about their own discomfort than about you. If you want to, reach out: "I've noticed some distance. I care about you. I'd like to stay connected, even if you're not sure what to say." And if they still don't come back, let them go. You deserve people who stay.

The Amateur Detective

- "Do you think it was your diet?"

- "Maybe it was stress?"

- "I read an article about deodorant..."

Nope. We're not turning this into a CSI episode. We're not assigning blame to broccoli or your old Victoria's Secret body spray. Say: "I'm more focused on healing than playing detective."

The Toxic Gift-Giver

- "Have you tried this magical supplement?"

- "Cut sugar. Cut dairy. Cut gluten. Cut happiness."

- "You should do yoga in a salt cave with vibrating goats."

Bless their crunchy little hearts. These folks mean well, but unless they have an MD or *are* the vibrating goat, their advice is best taken

147

with a grain of pink Himalayan salt. Try: "Thanks for thinking of me. I'm following the plan my doctor and I agreed on."

The Unsolicited Philosopher

- "Everything happens for a reason."

- "God doesn't give you more than you can handle."

- "This is making you stronger."

Hard pass. Sometimes, shitty things happen for absolutely no good reason. And telling someone they're becoming stronger while they're losing their hair, their energy, and their mind is just rude. A better approach would be to just say: "I'm sorry you're going through this. I'm here for you."

The Beauty Consultant

- "Your hair will grow back better than ever!"

- "You should try microblading."

- "Have you seen those eyebrow tattoos?"

Cool story, but maybe I just want to survive first. Some days, it takes everything to stand upright. Whether you're rocking a bald head or sticking on brows with Elmer's glue, your worth is not measured by your lashes. People can keep their beauty tips to themselves unless you *ask*.

Real Talk from Joyce: "Please... Don't Say That"

Joyce is one of the fiercest survivors I know, and she has exactly *zero* patience for unsolicited trauma dumps. Her biggest pet peeve was people calling to tell her about every sad cancer story they've ever heard.

"If you find out someone has cancer," she said, "please don't call to tell them about someone else who died from it."

Simple. Clear. True.

What *did* help her? Encouragement. Support. Acts of kindness. Not a play-by-play of your cousin's funeral.

A Mini Guide to What *To* Say

So now you're thinking, "Okay, I know what *not* to say. But what the hell *should* I say?"

Glad you asked.

- "I'm here for you."

- "This sucks. I'm so sorry."

- "I don't know what to say, but I'm not going anywhere."

- "Want company? Want space? Want memes?"

- "I'm going to the store. What can I grab for you?"

That's it. That's the magic. Show up. Don't try to fix it. Don't offer a solution. Just be present.

Bottom Line

You don't have to hold anyone else's awkwardness. You don't have to smile through ignorance or carry someone's fear in addition to your own. Let people show you who they are. And if they can't show up the way you need them to? That's not your fault.

This chapter of your life is hard enough. Don't waste your energy managing other people's discomfort.

Instead, surround yourself with those who don't flinch when you speak the hard truths. The ones who say, "I don't have the right words, but I've got snacks and time."

That's your people. That's your circle.

And trust me, they're worth their weight in gold.

You Get to Choose What You Share

You don't have to explain your treatment plan to every nosy neighbor. You don't have to justify your choices. You don't have to let people into your sacred space unless you want them there.

This is your life. Your story. Your body. You can answer, "How are you?" with "I'm still here." You can smile and say, "Not today." You can walk away from the conversation altogether.

⏱ Emotional Survival: You're Still in Control

In a world that feels like it's spinning off its axis, control becomes a kind of lifeline.

And you still have it. Not over the diagnosis, but over how you move through it.

If you're someone who calms your nerves by doing, give yourself a task: Start a journal. Keep a folder of appointments and test results. Make a list of people to tell and how you want to tell them. Write a letter to your future self, or to the child or grandchild who may one day need to understand what you walked through.

These small acts are more than coping. One day, your story may guide someone else in your family.

And when it does, they'll have your words, not just whispered memories.

🖌 Chapter Highlights

- **There's no perfect way to say "I have cancer."** Everyone processes and shares their diagnosis differently, and there's no script you have to follow.

- **Telling others is about connection and care.** Speaking your truth creates space for support and allows others to show up for you.

- **Choose your setting and words intentionally.** Share in quiet, safe environments and keep things simple and honest, without pressure to manage anyone else's emotions.

- **Offer people roles.** Help loved ones feel useful and included by giving them ways to support you.

- **Expect a range of reactions.** Not everyone will respond well. Some may offer support. Others may pull away. Neither response defines your value.

- **Telling your employer is personal and protected.** Share only what's necessary and explore your legal rights (FMLA, ADA, short-term disability).

- **You control your narrative.** You decide how much you share, with whom, and when. You don't owe anyone an explanation.

- **Not all responses will be helpful.** Be prepared for awkwardness, oversharing, toxic positivity, or silence. None of that is a reflection of you.

💟 **Key Takeaway**

You don't owe anyone a performance. Sharing your diagnosis is hard, but it can also open the door to connection, support, and even healing. You get to decide how your story is told.

"I don't want anybody to go through what I've been through."
— Kathy Bates; raised lymphedema awareness after double mastectomy

12
Brave Conversations With Little Hearts

When I was diagnosed, my oldest daughter was a teenager and my youngest was still in kindergarten. I don't remember the exact words I used to tell them. It's all a blur now, like trying to recall a dream after you've been awake for too long. But I do remember being honest. I took my time, sat with them, and did my best to reassure them that no matter what happened, we would figure it out together.

There wasn't a guidebook. No one handed me a script or sat me down to gently explain what words to use or which ones to avoid. I just followed my gut and tried not to scare them. It was clumsy and raw, but it was real. And sometimes real is the best we can offer.

Telling your child that you have cancer might be one of the hardest things you ever do. It's not only about finding the right words. You're shattering the part of their childhood that believes parents are invincible. The part that thinks mom can fix anything, do anything, *be* anything. And now, you're about to tell them something that makes the ground under their little feet feel less steady.

But here's what I want you to remember: kids are incredibly perceptive. They know when something isn't right, even if they don't have the words to name it. They feel the hush in the room, the glances exchanged between grownups. They see the extra doctor visits. They feel it in their bones when the house goes quiet in a new and unfamiliar way.

If you don't talk to them, they'll start filling in the blanks themselves. And what their imagination creates is almost always worse than the truth.

You don't need to explain everything. You don't need to walk them through the clinical terms or every possible outcome. But you do need to say something. Silence doesn't protect them. It just leaves them spinning in confusion and fear.

Speak in language they understand. Say the word: cancer. Let it be something they can name instead of fear in the shadows. You might say something like, *"Cancer means some of the cells in my body aren't doing their job right now. The doctors are helping me, and I'm doing everything I can to get better."*

And when the hard questions come, don't panic. It's okay not to have all the answers. Try, *"That's a really good question. I'm still learning the answer too, but I promise I'll tell you what I know when I know more."* That honesty, spoken gently, will build trust that lasts far beyond this season.

Reassure them of what won't change. Their home. Their routines. Your love. *"I might be more tired while I go through treatment. I might look different for a little while. But I'm still your mom. I still love you more than anything. And I'm still here."*

Younger kids especially need reminders that this isn't their fault. They might not say it, but it's not unusual for little ones to wonder if something they did somehow caused it. Let them know, *"This happened because of something in my body, not anything you said or did. And no matter what, I'm so proud to be your mom."*

If you're struggling to find a starting point, here's a simple one: *"The doctors found something in my body that doesn't belong. It's called cancer. I'm going to have some treatments to help me feel better. That might make me tired or change how I look, but I'm still me. And I'll always be here to love you."*

Your kids don't need a perfect explanation. They need you. Your presence. Your love. Your arms wrapped around them even on the hardest days. And in return, you might be surprised by the strength they offer back to you, in small and unexpected ways, like a coloring page left by your pillow or the way they snuggle a little closer at bedtime.

You are not alone in this. And neither are they.

✎ Melissa F., Diagnosed at 47

"I was raising two teenagers when I was diagnosed. It felt like the floor disappeared beneath us. My son started acting out in school. He'd never

154

done that before. My daughter withdrew completely, barely spoke at dinner. I realized they were terrified but didn't know how to say it. Once I sat them down, cried a little, and told them the truth, things shifted. Not overnight. But we started to talk again. I learned to say 'I don't know' when I didn't have answers, and that helped them trust me more than pretending to be strong all the time."

Melissa's experience is one that so many parents quietly share. Kids of all ages absorb stress like little emotional sponges. They notice the change in your energy, the extra appointments, the quiet crying in the bathroom. They don't need every medical detail, but they do need honesty. What they imagine in the absence of information is often even scarier than the truth.

📗 Age-Appropriate Conversations

You don't need to have a script, but it helps to speak in terms they understand.

For toddlers and preschoolers, keep it simple and concrete. Use words like "sick" and "medicine" and "tired." They live in the now, so focus on what's happening today, "Mommy needs to rest after her doctor visit," and repeat reassurances often. Their questions might seem random, but it's just how their brains process big change.

School-aged kids may want a bit more detail, especially about how your treatment will affect their routines. Will you still pick them up from practice? Will you be able to come to their recital? Let them know what to expect. They need structure and honesty more than sugar-coating.

Teenagers, though are a whole different animal. Some might ask deep, existential questions at midnight. Others will slam their doors and act like nothing is wrong. But don't be fooled, they're still watching, listening, and processing in their own time. Give them space, but don't assume their silence means they don't care. They do care. They just might not know how to show it yet.

Give Them Room to Speak

Not every child will respond right away. Some might ask a million questions. Others will say nothing at all. That's okay. What matters most is keeping the door open. You can gently check in with something like, "Do you want to talk about anything today?" or "Is there anything on your mind lately?" Then let them decide when and how they want to open up.

Sometimes they'll surprise you with a question you didn't expect, or with a quiet, unexpected hug. Sometimes they'll process things through art, play, or simply by being near you. Let that be enough.

Meet them with patience, honesty, and a steady presence. They don't need you to be invincible. They just need to know they're not alone in the uncertainty. And that kind of love is the most powerful medicine you can offer.

The Need for Reassurance

One of the hardest parts of being a parent with cancer isn't just what happens to your body. It's what your illness stirs up in them. Children are quiet collectors of emotion. They absorb everything: the shift in your energy, the whispered conversations, the worried looks exchanged over their heads, and without clear, loving reassurance, their imaginations can fill in the blanks with fears they're too young to explain.

Some children might silently wonder if they somehow caused your illness. Others might carry the terrifying question, "Are you going to die?" without ever saying the words out loud. That worry doesn't always come out in conversation. More often, it shows up in behavior. Tantrums that seem to come out of nowhere. Sudden clinginess. Mood swings. A child who tries so hard to be good it breaks your heart.

This is why reassurance matters. Why it needs to be spoken clearly, calmly, and more than once. Because they're not just hearing your words, they're watching your face, listening to your tone, trying to decode what's *really* going on.

Say it often:

"This is not your fault. You didn't cause this. Nothing you said or did made me sick."

"If I seem tired or grumpy, it's because of how my body feels, not because of anything you did."

"No matter what happens, you will always be cared for. You will never be alone."

You don't need to have every answer. You don't need to paint a picture that's too rosy or hide every hard truth. Just meet them where they are, and tell the truth with love.

Try something like:

"I can't promise everything will be easy. But I can promise this, we will face it together. You're not going through this alone, and neither am I."

That kind of honesty, when paired with comfort, becomes their anchor in the storm. And yours too.

Let Them Feel

Your child doesn't need a perfect parent right now. They just need permission to feel. Let them know it's okay to be sad, scared, mad, or confused. They don't have to pretend to be strong or act like everything's fine for your sake. Say it out loud: *"You're allowed to feel however you feel. And if it's too hard to talk to me about it, maybe we can find someone else to talk to. But I want you to know your feelings matter."* The gift of emotional permission, of not having to keep it together, is something they'll carry for the rest of their lives.

Keep Communication Open

This isn't going to be one big, brave conversation where everything gets wrapped up with a bow. This is a long road. An evolving one. Keep the lines of communication open, even when it's quiet. Even when they don't respond. Let them express themselves however they need to, through drawings, imaginary play, asking a million questions, or saying absolutely nothing. It all counts. Offer small, age-appropriate ways for them to be involved. Let them choose the movie on your rest days. Ask if they want to help decorate your calendar or check off medicine reminders. These tiny acts can make them feel included, grounded, and helpful.

📅 Predictability and Routine

When so much feels uncertain, routine becomes a lifeline. Children thrive on knowing what to expect. Let them know about schedule changes in advance whenever you can. "Aunt Jen will be picking you up from school this week," or "We might have dinner on the couch instead of the table for a while. Mom gets tired in the evenings." You might even consider using a visual calendar, checklist, or stickers so they can see what's coming next. Feeling a little more in control can bring a lot of comfort.

🖍️ Creative Outlets and the Coloring Book

For younger children, or kids who struggle to say how they feel, creative tools like drawing and coloring can become a bridge to conversation. Sometimes crayons are more honest than words. You can sit beside them, color quietly together, and give space for whatever needs to come out. You might be surprised what spills onto the page, or how much can be said without saying a thing.

😺 Teenagers Need You Too

Even if they roll their eyes, bury their heads in their phones, or act like they don't care, teenagers still need you. So much. Try saying something like, *"I know this is scary. It's scary for me too. But we're in this together. You don't have to talk about it all the time. Just know that you can always come to me. And I'll always be real with you."* They may not respond right away. But they'll remember that you said it. And they'll know they have a place to land when they're ready.

📐 Melissa L., Diagnosed at 54

"My son was in college when I told him I had cancer. He tried to be stoic, to act like it was no big deal. But then he texted me a few days later: 'Mom, I'm scared. But I've got you. Whatever you need.' That text is still saved in my phone. I didn't realize how much he was holding in until he finally let it out. It reminded me that even when they're grown, your kids still need you, and they still need to know it's okay to be scared."

💜 Helping Feels Like Healing

Letting kids help, even in small ways, can give them a powerful sense of control. Whether they're decorating your pill box, filling your water bottle, choosing a cozy blanket for treatment days, or drawing something silly for the fridge, it all matters. These little gestures remind them that they're not just helpless bystanders to something scary. It lets them know they're part of the team. Helping helps them feel strong. It gives them purpose in a moment that can feel incredibly confusing and out of control.

🍃 You Are Not Alone

And just like you need support, so do they. You don't have to walk this path alone, and neither do your children. There are picture books for little ones, teen support groups, school counselors, social workers, and therapists who specialize in helping kids navigate illness within the family. Reach out. Ask for help. Explore what's available in your community, or talk to your cancer center's social worker for resources.

Telling your child the truth won't break them. It will shape them. It will teach them how to walk through hard things with courage, honesty, and heart. Your example shows them what it means to stay connected, even when life turns upside down. And that, in the end, may be one of the most powerful gifts you can give.

✒️ Chapter Highlights

- Children are more perceptive than we think. They notice changes and will often create their own (scarier) explanations if not given the truth.

- Honest, age-appropriate conversations build trust. Use simple language, answer questions truthfully, and reassure often.

- Emotional reactions vary by age. Younger children may act out, teens may withdraw, but all responses are valid.

- Silence doesn't protect kids, it confuses them. Reassuring them that it's not their fault and that they will always be loved and cared for is essential.

- Include children in manageable ways. Small roles and routines help them feel connected and useful during a time when much feels out of their control.

- Ongoing communication is key. Check in regularly, offer outlets like play or art, and stay emotionally available, even when they seem distant.

🩶 Key Takeaway

Telling your child(ren) you have cancer doesn't mean you have every answer. You are giving them your presence, your honesty, and the reassurance that they are not alone in this journey.

If ever there is a tomorrow when we're not together,
there is something you must always remember:
You are braver than you believe,
Stronger than you seem,
And smarter than you think.
But the most important thing is, even if we're apart...
I'll always be with you.
—A.A. Milne (Christopher Robin)

13
Love, Loss, and Learning to be Seen Again

Cancer changed my body. But it also cracked my life wide open. In the beginning, people rallied. They dropped off casseroles, sent texts, and checked in. But eventually, they drifted back into the routines of their own lives. Meanwhile, I was still standing in the wreckage. Hair gone, body swollen from steroids, breasts tender and uneven from surgery. One of them had a four-inch scar where a chunk had been taken out. Nothing about me felt the same.

In my marriage, things got very quiet. We were both overwhelmed, but neither of us knew how to say it out loud. I didn't know how to let him in and he didn't know how to reach me. My body felt foreign. I avoided being seen. He withdrew. Our emotional distance turned into a physical distance as well.

Eventually, I learned he was having affairs. I was still trying to hold our family together while drowning under the weight of treatment, depression, and confusion. We were witnessing the collapse of everything we had built together. Our whole lives were wrapped up in lies, gaslighting, and denial. He wold twist things to make it look like my fault, even blaming me and saying I was cheating on him.

I reached the point where I couldn't argue with him any more. I didn't have fight left in me for him. I was frayed and unraveling. I had started drinking to cope. Then came the Tamoxifen. The mood swings hit hard. I felt like I was losing control of everything. My marriage. My mental health. My body. My future. My mind.

So I left. I walked away from our house. I didn't fight for half of his military retirement, even after ten years of marriage. Even though I had left the military six years earlier to care for our family while he continued in the service. I let the kids stay with him, because I had nowhere to go. He cut me off from our joint bank account, and I couldn't afford a lawyer or a place to live because he was having child support taken out of my meager paychecks. For a time, I lived out of my Jeep with my dog and a trash bag full of clothes.

That was my rock bottom.

Finding Clarity in the Chaos

And yet, looking back now, I understand more than I did then. I blamed him for the cheating, the lies, the way he seemed to move on so easily. But I also know that I wasn't okay either. I didn't make things easy because I was spiraling, and he didn't know how to deal with it. That doesn't excuse what he did. But it helps me make peace with the full picture.

We both contributed to the breaking of that marriage.

If I could go back, I would have begged for therapy for myself, for us, for our kids. I would have told someone I was drowning. I would have stopped pretending I could handle it alone. Maybe the marriage wouldn't have survived, but we could have separated without as much damage. Maybe my children wouldn't have had to watch everything between us fall apart in silence.

So I'm telling you now: Don't wait until you're at your breaking point. If your relationship is bending under the weight of cancer, ask for help. Fight for your connection with honesty, softness, and vulnerability. Your body may have changed. Your needs may feel unfamiliar and intimacy may feel complicated. But that doesn't mean you are broken or unlovable.

It just means you're a person going through a devastating time in your life.

Please don't try to carry all of this alone. There is support out there for individuals, couples, and families. It's okay to need it. It's okay to want it. And it's okay to ask for it, even if you don't know exactly what you need. You are worth saving, no matter what's been lost.

Joyce's Story: Holding On Together

Joyce's marriage didn't fall apart. In fact, she says their relationship became stronger. That doesn't mean it was easy, but it means they were intentional about talking and sharing. They cried together. They laughed in hospital rooms and her husband made her feel beautiful,

162

even when she felt anything but. He learned about side effects and showed up in quiet, meaningful ways. She told me they didn't pretend it was all fine; they just stayed honest, even when things got messy.

"We didn't have the perfect marriage," she said. "But we were willing to sit in the hard stuff together. We figured it out."

It's important to share both sides. Not every relationship breaks under the pressure. And if yours doesn't, that's something to treasure and nurture.

When Intimacy Becomes Complicated

After cancer, your relationship with your own body changes in ways you never imagined. Scars appear where smooth skin used to be. Your shape may shift, gaining or losing weight in places you never expected. Hair disappears, ports are placed, your skin may feel tender or numb. These changes aren't merely physical, they're seriously emotional. Each new difference in your reflection becomes another reminder that life is not what it once was. You look in the mirror and sometimes feel like a stranger is staring back at you. There's a particular kind of grief that comes from losing the version of yourself you once knew so intimately. A quiet ache that lingers in the unfamiliar.

And eventually, the question rises, softly, uncertainly, painfully: how can I let someone else see me like this, when I don't even recognize myself?

It can be incredibly difficult to trust someone to respond with kindness and love when you haven't fully processed your own feelings yet. And while it might not be spoken aloud, your partner may be grieving too. Not just the changes to your body, but the way your closeness feels different now. Sometimes, they're afraid to touch you, not out of rejection or lack of desire, but because they're unsure what's okay anymore. They don't want to hurt you physically, or emotionally. So they pull back, and then you do too. You both tiptoe around the pain, trying to protect each other, and in the process, the quiet space between you grows wider. The connection you both need so much, starts to feel unreachable.

What once came so naturally between you now feels impossible. The brush of a hand. A soft kiss. The way your body used to respond to touch. Now you're navigating fatigue, brain fog, hormonal shifts, mood swings, and side effects you were never warned about. You might be experiencing vaginal dryness or painful intercourse. Your libido might have packed a bag and walked off without so much as a goodbye. Or maybe you're simply too exhausted to even consider intimacy at all.

But just know that you are not broken. You are healing. And healing doesn't mean snapping back into who you were before. It means gently rediscovering what feels good, what doesn't, what you need, what you want. That process might feel awkward at first, but awkward doesn't mean wrong. It means you're showing up. It means you're trying. And that kind of bravery is beautiful.

There are tools that can help with the physical aspects: vaginal moisturizers, lubricants, pelvic floor therapy, even prescription medications. But sometimes, the most powerful step you can take is simply being honest. Start with your doctor. Ask the questions that make you squirm. Talk about the discomfort, the confusion, the loss of desire. Trust me, they've heard it all. You won't shock them, and you won't be judged. Their job is to support you.

Then, when you're ready, talk to your partner. You don't need a polished speech. You don't need all the right words. Just open the door, even if it's only a crack. Say, "This is hard for me to talk about, but I need to try." Or, "Can we be real with each other about what this feels like, even if it's messy?" Because intimacy isn't just about sex. It's about trust. It's about allowing yourself to be fully seen and still feel safe. It's about quiet moments, eye contact, closeness, and emotional safety wrapped in physical tenderness.

You're allowed to want touch. You're allowed to take things slowly. To ask for softness. To say no. To say yes. To change your mind. You are allowed to explore your body again with curiosity, gentleness, and compassion. The more you communicate, the easier it becomes to rebuild connection, not just physically, but emotionally. And when you let someone see the most vulnerable parts of you, and they stay, and they hold you with love, you realize that intimacy never left. It just needed a new way to begin.

You deserve that kind of love. You deserve to be held, not just by someone else, but by yourself, with grace and patience and care. You are still whole. You are still beautiful. You are still worthy of joy.

✒ Melissa F., Diagnosed at 47

It started with a dimple. Just a subtle indentation on my right breast. Barely noticeable, but enough to spark a gut feeling. I called my doctor right away and scheduled a mammogram. The results came back: "large dense breasts," nothing to worry about. So the next year, I skipped my appointment. I didn't want to waste anyone's time. That decision haunted me.

By the time I returned for another mammogram, something had changed. This time, they weren't so confident. A biopsy followed, and that's when the world tilted: I had stage 2, hormone-positive breast cancer. I was 47 years old, married, and raising two teenage kids. But in that moment, I was just a daughter, terrified of leaving my children without a mother, the way I had lost mine at 25. That pain, that absence, still lived in me. I couldn't imagine doing that to my children.

I chose a double mastectomy. Some might say it doesn't guarantee anything, but for me, it brought peace. I didn't want the constant fear of recurrence hanging over me. I wanted it gone. All of it.

What I didn't expect was how utterly alone I would feel. My husband grew cold and distant. One day he told me he couldn't look at me the same after surgery. I stopped looking in the mirror. I felt mutilated. I felt ugly. I didn't go out. I didn't want to be seen, not by strangers, not by people who loved me, not even by myself.

Reconstruction was a long process, but I clung to it because I needed *something* to help me feel normal again. Something to pull me out of that dark place. I started taking care of myself, eating better, moving more, applying for jobs. I got hired. I started smiling again. And wouldn't you know it, my husband decided he wanted to work things out. But I looked at him and said, "You didn't love me at my lowest. You don't get to love me at my best."

I'm four years past diagnosis now. Divorced. Healing. Still on anastrozole. Still figuring it out. But I no longer hide from my scars.

165

I'm proud of them. My new boobs are a C cup. Bras are optional now, and any woman would know, that part's kind of fun.

I was consumed by the fire… and I rose like a phoenix.

💔 The Grief No One Talks About

One woman told me, "No one warned me how much I would mourn the loss of my fertility."

For younger women especially, this part of the journey can feel like a silent heartbreak. You may not have even known you were ready to think about kids. Maybe you had plans, maybe you didn't. But the second cancer enters the room, that choice, that possibility, gets swept off the table. And suddenly, you're grieving something you might not have even realized you were holding onto.

It's the grief of a door closing. A future changing and options being taken away. A version of you that may never exist.

And it's not always about whether you *can* still have children. It's about how quickly that decision was taken away from you. About how rushed and medicalized something so personal became. You're told to focus on survival, and you do, but quietly, in the background, this ache builds into a mountain. It shows up when your friends announce pregnancies. When you see baby clothes in a store. When your partner holds a child and something inside you flinches.

And the worst part is that most people don't even know to ask about it. They don't realize it's one of the things that can happen. So you carry it alone.

If you're partnered, this might be something you both mourn, or something you experience differently. Maybe your partner doesn't fully understand the depth of that loss, or maybe they're trying to be strong for you while quietly hurting too. These conversations can be hard. But bringing them into the light is part of healing. You're allowed to talk about it. You're allowed to cry about it. You're allowed to feel it *all:* anger, sadness, confusion, guilt, even relief, if that's part of your truth.

If you're single, this can feel like another kind of loss. The imagined family. The timeline. The dating conversations that suddenly feel impossibly complicated.

None of this is simple. But here's what I want you to know:
You are not alone.
You are still worthy of love, of partnership, of closeness.
And your grief is not too much. It's valid, and it matters.

If you're reading this before treatment, talk to your doctor about fertility preservation. Even if you're not sure what you want yet. You deserve options. You deserve time.

And if you've already come through treatment and this door has closed, please hear this with love: It's not your fault. You were trying to save your own life. That is not a failure. That is the fiercest kind of strength.

You are still whole. You are still you.
Even in the ache. Even in the absence.
You are still enough.

🚀 Rebuilding Connection

Reconnecting after cancer doesn't always look the way it used to. And that's okay. If you're partnered, maybe intimacy right now isn't about sex at all. Maybe it's long hugs in the kitchen. Laying close under a blanket with the TV on low. Taking a shower together, not for arousal, but to feel the closeness of warm water and safe hands. Sometimes, it's holding each other through tears. Or laughter. Or silence.

If you're single, this can feel even more vulnerable. The idea of letting someone new see your scars, both physical and emotional, might feel like too much. But please hear this: your worth is not measured by your breasts or your libido. You are still deserving of love, affection, and desire.

And you don't have to figure it all out alone.

There are people and resources out there who specialize in helping survivors rebuild their sense of self. Sex therapists, especially those who understand cancer's impact, can help you navigate these changes with compassion and practical tools. Support groups offer a space to share and listen without shame. And sometimes, even a well-timed podcast or book can make you feel seen in ways you didn't expect.

Andrea, a fellow survivor, told me, *"I had to go through a whole process of seeing myself as beautiful. Not just physically, but spiritually and emotionally. But I still grieve the old me sometimes. The me before scars and stretch marks and chemo hair."*

God, yes. That grief for our old selves. We don't talk about it enough. But it's there, just under the surface: sometimes loud, sometimes whispering.

If you're struggling, it doesn't mean you've failed. You've been through something huge, and like any significant time in your life, you'll need space for healing with time, patience, and care.

You're not broken. And there is hope, even here.
Even in the difficult times and quiet places.
Even when you feel miles away from your old self.
Take small steps and give yourself some grace to find your way back to you.

Let this be a reminder that your story isn't over, it's unfolding. And connection, in all its forms, is still waiting for you.

✍ Melissa L., Diagnosed at 54

My name is Melissa L., and I was 54 when I was diagnosed with Stage 1 HER2+ mucinous carcinoma, because even my cancer had to be extra. I wasn't entirely surprised. I'd had years of mammograms with that same spot marked as "something to watch." It felt like it had been playing hide-and-seek for sixteen years and finally decided to show itself.

I started with chemo and immunotherapy, followed by surgery and radiation. It wasn't easy, especially the TCHP chemo. That stuff flattened me. But one moment during treatment changed everything for me.

I was walking through the infusion center after a port draw, heading to my oncologist appointment, when I saw another woman sitting in a chair, crying. Her husband was next to her, trying so hard to comfort her, but I knew those tears. I recognized the kind of pain that can't be comforted with words.

I gave her a little space, then quietly walked over, looked her in the eye, and said, "We've got this. Just breathe. One day at a time." She didn't say anything at first. She just reached out and held my hand, and we sat there for a few quiet moments together. That's when I realized that there's something really powerful about being seen by someone who truly understands. Support from family and friends is wonderful, but there's a different kind of peace that comes from standing eye to eye with someone else who's in the fire too.

That moment changed how I moved through treatment. From then on, I made it my mission to look for the people who needed a smile, a laugh, or just someone to sit with. I became the comic relief in the infusion center. I called myself a "pole dancer" any time I had to shuffle around with my IV pole. I made sarcastic comments about being roasted medium rare during radiation. And to my surprise, others started laughing with me. Nurses began using the "pole dancer" line. Patients got up and did a little spin as they headed to the bathroom.

I realized that humor was a kind of medicine. Connection was a kind of healing. And showing up for each other was the most real thing we could do.

Cancer changed me. I give myself more grace now. I don't waste time chasing people who don't show up for me. I know what really matters. Laughter. Kindness. Connection. These are the things that carried me through, and now I try to carry them forward, every chance I get.

🔔 Prosthetics, Bras, and Being Seen Again

Your body is different now. Whether you had a lumpectomy, a mastectomy, chose reconstruction, or decided to go flat, there's a shift. You see it in the mirror. You feel it every time you take a shower. You notice the way your clothes fit. And sometimes, that change hits you like a punch to the gut.

169

Some women prefer not to undergo reconstruction, and breast prosthetics can offer a comfortable and empowering alternative to reconstruction. They can help restore symmetry under clothing, bring back a little confidence, and add a sense of normalcy when everything else feels unfamiliar. Some are soft foam forms. Others are silicone, weighted to mimic the natural feel. Some slip into a bra, others adhere directly to the skin. Fortunately, there are plenty of options, and there's no one right or wrong choice. Only what feels right for you.

Some women wear prosthetics every day. Some pull them out only for special occasions. Some tuck them in a drawer and never look back. And some walk proudly, beautifully flat. All of it is valid. You get to decide what makes you feel whole.

Post-surgical bras are a different world from the lacy underthings you might've worn before. They're softer. Front-closing. Wire-free. Designed with healing in mind. Some have built-in pockets for prosthetics. Others just offer gentle support where you need it most. And when you find one that actually makes you feel good, it can be a surprisingly powerful thing.

Then there's hair. Losing it can feel like shedding a piece of your identity. For some, it's the hardest part. For others, it's strangely freeing. And when it grows back, it might come back curlier, thicker, even a new color. It becomes one more layer in the story of becoming someone new.

While you wait, you have options. Wigs that let you recreate your old look or try something completely new. Scarves and wraps that turn your head into a canvas of expression. Soft, cozy hats for warmth and comfort. Or maybe nothing at all, just your brave, beautiful bare head.

Some women choose to reclaim their bodies with adornments like tattoos over scars, new piercings, bold clothes that celebrate instead of conceal. Others lean into quiet softness, comfort and privacy. There is no one way to rediscover yourself. Just a thousand small choices, all leading you to your new self.

And here's what matters most: you are allowed to grieve the body you had. And you are also allowed to love the one you have now.

You are allowed to want to feel beautiful again.

You are allowed to define what beauty means on your terms.

You are still worthy of desire. Of tenderness. Of joy, in whatever form that takes.

So go slow. Try new things. Laugh at the awkwardness. Cry when it hurts. Give yourself permission to feel everything. And remember, learning to love your body again doesn't mean loving every inch of it, every day. It just means choosing not to abandon yourself.

✔ Chapter Highlights

- Cancer often brings emotional and physical changes that can quietly erode intimacy and connection in relationships.

- Infidelity and emotional withdrawal may stem from unspoken grief, unmet needs, and mutual overwhelm, not just malice.

- Survivors often experience body image struggles, loss of libido, and confusion around physical touch or sexual closeness.

- Tools like pelvic floor therapy, lubricants, and honest conversations with partners and doctors can support healing.

- Fertility grief is a real and often unacknowledged loss for younger survivors. It deserves space and compassion.

- Reconnection takes time, honesty, vulnerability, and the willingness to explore new forms of closeness.

💜 Key Takeaway

Your body may feel different. Your needs may feel unfamiliar. But you are still whole, still worthy of tenderness, desire, and love. Intimacy isn't gone—it's simply asking to be rediscovered with care.

I will not rescue you, for you are not powerless.
I will not fix you, for you are not broken.
I will walk with you through the darkness,
as you remember your light.
— *L.R. Knost*

14

The Reality of Early Menopause

I had my first hot flash at thirty-one, and it wasn't subtle. It hit me like a wave of fire rising from the inside out, as if someone had struck a match somewhere behind my ribcage and it spread instantly to my skin. One minute I was folding laundry in the living room, completely fine, and the next, I was drenched in sweat, flushed bright red, and peeling off layers like I was trying to escape my own body. My hair stuck to the back of my neck, and I stood there, staring at the ceiling fan like it was personally failing me. It felt like my body had betrayed me, and I didn't even know what to call it yet.

No one tells you that menopause might come crashing into your life when you're still young enough to have babies. When your kids are little and your plans are still unfolding. I thought I had time to decide if I wanted more children. Time to explore my options. But chemo didn't just mess with my cycles. It brought everything to a screeching halt, and it did so without warning. There was no gentle transition or slow fade like I had always imagined menopause to be. It didn't wait for my body to be ready. It just barged in, uninvited, and took over.

Marissa was just 28 when she was told cancer treatment might leave her infertile. "I didn't even have a boyfriend at the time," she said, "but I still cried like someone had stolen something from me. I hadn't decided if I wanted kids, but I wanted the chance to decide for myself. That choice being taken from me broke something I didn't know was fragile."

Before treatment, I had regular cycles and hopes for the future. Afterward, all of that changed. My eyebrows thinned out, my skin lost its glow, I developed hemorrhoids I wasn't expecting, and I stared down an empty calendar where my period used to be. It was disorienting, like someone had hit fast-forward on a part of life I wasn't ready for yet.

Kim considered preserving her fertility, but the logistics were overwhelming. "I was already drowning in appointments when they brought up egg freezing," she said. "The cost. The hormones. The timing. I didn't have the energy to fight for something I wasn't even sure I'd use. But walking away from that option felt like giving up on a whole future I hadn't even dreamed yet."

And now, years later, I find myself going through it again, this time the natural version of menopause, and it feels almost like my body remembers. Like it's already tired of the fight and is just going through the motions one more time. The hot flashes, the joint aches, the sleepless nights, they all returned, only this time, there's a quiet familiarity that makes it even more frustrating.

Danielle put it bluntly: "Hot flashes. Mood swings. Vaginal dryness. The joy of being 35 going on 55. Nobody tells you that chemo can flip the switch and shove you into menopause overnight. I wasn't ready for that."

Menopause is hard at any age, but when it's forced by treatment, it feels different. There's no grace period, no adjustment time. It's like waking up one day and realizing a piece of your identity has been taken without your consent. You didn't get to choose this. You didn't even get a warning.

Even if you weren't planning on having more children, or never wanted any at all, the loss of making your own choice still stings. There's grief in losing the ability to decide. There's grief in your body feeling like it aged ten years overnight. And there's grief in looking at yourself in the mirror and wondering who that person is staring back at you, flushed and tired, her clothes clinging to skin that suddenly feels like it doesn't fit quite right anymore.

But even in the middle of all of this, you're still you. You're still capable of finding comfort, of reclaiming your body in new ways, of stepping into this next chapter with courage.

You didn't choose this version of menopause, but you are surviving it. And that matters more than anyone realizes.

🐛 What the Doctors Call It (and Why It Still Hurts)

Chemotherapy and hormone therapy can abruptly halt ovarian function, leading to either temporary or permanent menopause. For some, menstruation returns after treatment. For others, it never does.

In medical terms, it's called treatment-induced menopause or chemotherapy-induced ovarian failure. But those words don't quite capture the emotional weight of it. This isn't just a pause in periods. It's making big changes to your body that maybe you weren't prepared for.

🔥 Symptoms: It's Not Just Hot Flashes

You know what's really fun? Having your estrogen snatched away like a toddler yanking a toy out of your hand. One day you're learning to navigate cancer, and the next you're sweating through your sheets at 2 a.m., picking a fight with your toaster, crying because someone looked at you wrong, and Googling "Can you die from hot flashes?" just to be sure.

This isn't the gentle gliding descent of natural menopause, that takes years to develop and change your body. Oh no. This is a hormonal cliff dive with no parachute, no warning, and definitely no soft landing. It's like your body got the memo about menopause and said, "Bet. Let's do it all at once, immediately, and with no grace whatsoever."

Suddenly you're managing a chaotic cocktail of symptoms that no one properly prepared you for. Hot flashes so aggressive you feel like you're being slow-roasted from the inside out. Mood swings that turn you from weepy to homicidal in seconds. Vaginal dryness that feels like your lady parts are made out of sandpaper. Brain fog that has you walking into rooms and forgetting your own name. And your joints sound like you're popping popcorn every time you stand up.

And let's not even start on the sleep. Or rather, the lack thereof. You take forever to fall asleep. You toss, you turn, you sweat through your third set of sheets. You wake up at 2am only to lie there wide awake, listening to your spouse happily dreaming, and seriously consider the ramifications of smothering them with a pillow, until your alarm goes off and you're supposed to act like a functioning human being. Cute.

But here's where it really gets cruel: while your body is undergoing an identity crisis, you're also emotionally unraveling. There's grief. Real, guttural, soul-deep grief. Especially if you hadn't finished having children, or hadn't even started. It's losing an entire imagined future, ripped away before you even got to decide if you wanted it. No one tells you how much that'll hurt. Or how furious you might feel.

Lauren J., diagnosed at 33, described it perfectly: "It wasn't just my period that stopped. It was everything. The decision to have a baby was taken away from me before I even got to make it. And nobody warned me how angry I'd feel. I wasn't just sad, I was furious. Like my body betrayed me again after everything I'd already given."

It's one more thing cancer took without asking.

So if you're out here feeling like you've been hit by a hormonal freight train, questioning your sanity, annoyed with everyone around you, or raging at husband because the ceiling fan isn't cooling you fast enough, please know this isn't you. This is the aftermath no one talks about. This is the price tag hanging off the bright pink "you survived!" balloon.

And it's okay to be mad about it. It's also okay to laugh through your tears and swear at your ovaries. This is hard. And utterly ridiculous. And real. And you're allowed to feel every messy, complicated bit of it.

Even if your estrogen isn't coming back, your sense of humor can stick around. And some days, that might be the only thing that saves you.

Why Are More Young Women Going Through This?

Breast cancer in younger women isn't the rare unicorn it used to be. In fact, it's showing up more often than ever before. Recent studies are confirming what many of us already suspected; diagnosis rates are rising in women under 50, particularly those in their 30s and early 40s. That means more and more women are being shoved into early menopause, not by biology, but by chemo, surgery, and medication, right in the middle of what's supposed to be the prime of their lives.

This isn't a slow transition marked by a few skipped periods and a drawer full of fans and herbal teas. This is a hard stop. One minute, you're managing your cycle and planning your future. The next, you're hemorrhaging estrogen, waking up in sweat-soaked sheets, and wondering how you got thrown into the menopause club before you were done having kids, or figuring out if you even wanted them at all.

Everyone seems to have a theory about why this is happening, and yet no one can seem to pin it down. Theories include environmental toxins, endocrine disruptors in your shampoo, plastic in your coffee lids, processed food, earlier puberty, later pregnancies, obesity, genetics, alcohol, chronic stress, or maybe just better detection. Take your pick. Every time you turn around, there's a new headline blaming something else. Meanwhile, more and more women are losing their breasts, their ovaries, and their fertility before their fortieth birthday, and the only real answer we seem to get is a collective shrug from the medical community.

And it's infuriating. It feels like no one is connecting the dots while the numbers keep climbing. We're living in a system more interested in pink ribbon slogans, awareness themes, and fundraising campaigns, than actual prevention or answers.

But this isn't only about how annoying hot flashes can be. It's about fertility. About family planning and the very real grief of losing the option to choose when or whether to have children. It's about facing bone loss, heart risks, memory issues, mood swings, and body changes that make you feel like you've aged decades overnight. It's about being handed a generic menopause pamphlet in a cold doctor's office while your friends are posting gender reveals and bump updates on Instagram.

It's about trying to laugh when someone jokes about "finally being done with their period" while you're quietly mourning yours, and everything it represented.

This is the part of cancer that hits below the surface. It messes with your identity, your relationships, your sense of time and possibility. It can eat away at your hope. And it deserves more than silence and guesswork. It deserves attention. Advocacy. And a hell of a lot more compassion for what it actually means to be a young woman walking through this fire.

💔 The Hidden Grief of Early Menopause

There is grief here. It doesn't wear black or announce itself with a funeral, but it lives in your bones. It's in the quiet heartache of unrealized plans. The guilt of not wanting to have sex when everything hurts. The flash of resentment when you see a baby shower invitation land in your inbox.

You feel older than your peers, alienated from the rhythm of what's supposed to be "normal."

🔧 Real Tools That Actually Help

Body support: Layered clothing and cooling sheets became my tools for survival. Regular movement, even if it is just slow stretching, help your joints feel less like gravel. Keeping a damp washcloth in the fridge or small ice packs in the freezer, and pressing them to your neck or chest when a flash hits also helps tremendously.

Medical support: You can talk to your doctor about vaginal estrogen. Research antidepressants and gabapentin, and talk with your doctor about them. Learn about pelvic floor therapy and take it seriously. You have to stop pretending it didn't matter and start advocating for your comfort.

Sarai P., diagnosed at 41, described her experience like this: "I felt like a ghost of myself. Like my body still existed but my desire had evaporated. I was embarrassed to talk about it, until my oncologist mentioned pelvic floor therapy. That one sentence changed everything. I wasn't broken. I just needed help."

Mental and emotional support: Let yourself journal, and don't hold back on your thoughts and feelings. Cry when you need to, and surround yourself with people that let you be yourself. Find spaces where you can say, "This sucks," without someone jumping in with their toxic positivity. Give yourself permission to grieve what you've lost and to sit in the confusion of who you are now. Most importantly, speak up. Tell your doctors, your loved ones, your friends what you need.

178

You Are Not Alone

There's nothing weak about feeling unsteady. There's nothing wrong with mourning what was taken from you. You're not less of a woman. You're not broken. You're changed.

Early menopause from cancer treatment doesn't just change your body, it can shake your sense of identity and future. But with honesty, support, and care, you can reclaim your voice, your power, and your life.

Chapter Highlights

- Chemotherapy and hormone therapy can lead to temporary or permanent early menopause, known as treatment-induced menopause.

- Symptoms can include hot flashes, insomnia, mood swings, vaginal dryness, joint pain, and brain fog.

- The emotional impact is significant: grief, body image changes, intimacy issues, and a sense of lost control are common.

- Early menopause can affect fertility, identity, and future plans.

- The incidence of breast cancer in younger women is rising due to a combination of possible factors, including environmental toxins, delayed childbirth, lifestyle choices, and better screening.

- Coping strategies include lifestyle adjustments (cooling products, movement), medical support (medications, pelvic floor therapy), and emotional care (therapy, journaling, survivor groups).

- Open communication with your care team and self-advocacy are crucial for managing this phase of treatment.

🤍 Key Takeaway

Early menopause from cancer treatment doesn't just change your body, it can shake your sense of identity and future. But with honesty, support, and care, you can reclaim your voice, your power, and your life.

"She is clothed in strength and dignity, and she laughs without fear of the future."
— Proverbs 31:25

15
Feeding the Body, Honoring the Fight

During treatment, eating became one of the hardest tasks I faced. Nothing tasted the way it used to. My mouth always felt like it was coated in metal. Some days even the smell of food was enough to turn my stomach. But I knew I needed fuel. I needed to make it through chemo, or the drive to radiation, or simply to stay upright.

Kristie said it best: "I couldn't even *think* about meat without gagging. The smell of anything cooking made me nauseous, and I basically lived on toast, tea, and frozen grapes. People kept telling me to 'just eat,' but nothing felt safe."
That was it exactly. You want to eat. You try. But your body suddenly treats food like an enemy, and no one else seems to get it.

One of the best tips I ever got came before chemo even started: Don't eat your favorite foods. At first, it sounded ridiculous. Why not eat what brings you comfort? But it turns out, it's brilliant advice. Chemo has a way of turning everything you eat into a sensory nightmare: metallic, medicinal, strange. And those new, awful associations don't go away when treatment ends. By steering clear of my comfort foods, I protected them. I didn't turn tacos into trauma. I didn't ruin my love for strawberries or my favorite ice cream. I kept those things sacred, and years later, I'm so grateful I did.

Nutrition during cancer has nothing to do with kale or green juice. Forget macros, clean eating, or trying to get it "just right." The focus is just on doing what you can to make it through. Some days, that looked like a single spoonful of applesauce and half a saltine. Other days, it meant lying in the dark, sipping broth, and letting someone else carry the weight for a while.

Elena shared something that really stayed with me. "I used to obsess over dieting, but cancer made me realize how important it is to *feed* your body, not punish it. I started making smoothies, eating more color, and listening to what my body needed instead of what the scale said." There's something sacred about that shift. Food stops being a measurement of worth and becomes a way to care for yourself with tenderness and intention.

Sometimes, self-care wasn't pretty. It meant saying no. Perhaps canceling plans. Sometimes it was letting the floor stay messy and the laundry pile up. It meant giving myself permission to rest without guilt.

Your job during treatment isn't to impress anyone. Your job is to make it through this journey. To be kind to yourself. To meet each day with grace when you can, and forgiveness when you can't.

The Myth of Prevention

Before we dive into nutrition and lifestyle in the next section, I want to hit pause and talk about something really important.

Not long ago, I asked a breast cancer Facebook group, "If there were a book about breast cancer, what would you want it to include?" I expected the usual answers: more clarity around medical options, encouragement to let go of the pressure to be strong all the time, stories that felt hopeful and real.

But one woman said this: *"I wish there had been a preventative book. Something I could've read that might've helped me avoid getting cancer in the first place."*

Reading that hit me harder than I expected. Seventeen years into remission, and those words still tugged something loose. I started wondering: *Wait... did I miss something? Could I have prevented this?* And just like that, I was spiraling. Wondering what I could have done differently. Questioning if I had caused my own cancer. Even now, even after all this time, it got to me.

And I want to stop you before you go down the same road that I did.

You're going to hear a lot of noise out there. Articles. Documentaries. Podcasts. Wellness influencers. Strangers on the internet. Some of it will be helpful. A lot of it won't. You'll hear what you "should" have done. What someone else swears would've saved you. You'll hear about magic diets and detoxes and supplement stacks, and some of it might make you feel like maybe this is your fault.

First, people need to keep their opinions to themselves. Don't be afraid to set your boundaries and let them know you're doing just fine without them telling you everything they think you could have or should have done. Opinions are like ass holes. You know the rest.

Second, and this one is very important, so I'll say this as clearly as I can:

You did not cause your cancer.

Yes, there are choices that can support your immune system, like eating more plants, getting better sleep, drinking less, managing stress. All of that can help. But let's be honest: people who do everything "right" still get cancer. And people who never touch a vegetable live to ninety without a hitch. Cancer doesn't care how good you've been. It doesn't keep score, and it sure as hell doesn't play fair.

The next section isn't here to hand out gold stars or make you feel like you dropped the ball. It's not a checklist to measure your worth or how hard you've tried. It's a starting place. Just simple things you might try if you're looking for ways to feel a little stronger or more like yourself again. These are just things you can try because feeling better is something you absolutely deserve.

If walking for twenty minutes makes you feel more like yourself again, let's do that. If eating a rainbow-colored plate of veggies helps your digestion or your mood, great. If skipping that third glass of wine gives you a clearer head in the morning, awesome.

But none of it is about fixing something broken.

You're not broken, you're healing.

This isn't about the life you had before cancer. It's about the life you're living now, and how to best care for the person who's still standing.

Nutrition During Treatment

Category	Tips & Examples
Hydration	Aim for 8–10 cups/day: water, broths, herbal teas

183

Electrolyte Balance	Use coconut water, electrolyte tablets, low-sugar drinks like Nuun or Liquid I.V.
Easy-to-Digest Meals	Choose soft or bland foods: toast, bananas, scrambled eggs
Protein Sources	Chicken, tofu, yogurt, beans, nut butter, protein shakes
High-Calorie Foods	Include avocado, olive oil, nuts, and comfort food when needed
Foods to Avoid	Avoid raw meat, unwashed produce, alcohol, and strong spices
Managing Taste Changes	Use plastic utensils, suck citrus, rinse mouth with baking soda water
Managing Nausea	Eat small meals, use ginger or peppermint, ask for nausea meds
Electrolyte Support	Add powders like Liquid I.V., limit caffeine if dizzy
Managing Dizziness	Stand up slowly, snack on pretzels, consult your doctor if ongoing
Constipation Relief	Stay hydrated, eat prunes, consider stool softeners if needed
Immune-Boosting Foods	Include citrus, berries, leafy greens, garlic, nuts, and green tea

Cancer turns nutrition into something entirely different. Some days, you eat what you can. Other days, you're just trying to get through the next bite without feeling sick. Your goal right now should be to just find ways to provide hydration and nutrition to your body in order to heal and keep moving forward.

A helpful resource that many survivors have leaned on is a book called *Cancer Nutrition and Me: From Diagnosis to Healing* by McBarry Joel. In this book, the author doesn't assume you're a nutritionist or that you're trying to be perfect. It meets you where you are and gives gentle advice about how to care for your body when food is the last thing on your mind. It offers strategies for when you're nauseous, emotionally drained, or just too tired to chew. If you want a book that supports you like a friend while still giving you science you can trust, this one may be worth looking into.

Why Food Matters — Even When It's Hard

Your body is doing hard, invisible work. Whether it's processing chemo, healing from surgery, or just trying to stay upright through radiation, your system is under a lot of pressure. Good nutrition can help reduce fatigue, improve recovery, lessen the sting of side effects, and keep your strength up for whatever comes next. That doesn't mean you have to eat kale and quinoa every day. Sometimes nutrition is soup from a can or half a banana. It still counts.

Staying hydrated helps your body flush out toxins. Protein helps you hold onto muscle. Gentle fiber can ease digestive struggles. And sometimes, just managing to get one good bite down is enough.

Gentle Meals for Gentle Days

While undergoing treatment, there were days when all I could manage was applesauce or broth. So I started batch cooking on good days. Soups and casseroles portioned out into freezer bags became my lifeline. When I couldn't stand long enough to cook, I could heat something with the push of a button. And when that wasn't an option, I had a drawer full of saltines, instant oatmeal, pudding cups, and bananas.

I found that smaller bowls helped me eat more. A full dinner plate felt overwhelming, but a teacup full of something soft felt manageable. And if all I could get down was a frozen waffle? Well, that would have to be enough for now.

Dining Out Without the Pressure

Restaurants can feel overwhelming when your system is delicate. I found myself drawn to simple meals: grilled chicken, baked potatoes, plain toast, broth-based soups. If something came too seasoned or greasy, I didn't hesitate to ask for a change. And I stopped being afraid to say, "This is a medical thing." Most people are happy to help, but you have to let them know how.

I stayed away from raw bars and buffets, and when getting fast food, I requested that my food be made fresh, not something sitting under a heat lamp. There is less opportunity for bacteria to grow that way.

185

Knowing my immune system couldn't handle the risk, I felt safer asking that the food be cooked fresh. That one quiet decision probably saved me more than once.

Letting Others Help With Food

It took courage to say out loud, "I can't eat that right now." But being honest helped others help me. I started suggesting restaurants with smoothies or soft foods. When friends offered to bring something over, I stopped saying "Oh, anything," and started asking for what I really needed. Items like homemade broth, soft banana bread, gentle soup sat so much better on my delicate system during that time.

Food as Support for Side Effects

Treatment comes with a long list of side effects, and some of them show up right in your kitchen. For nausea, small frequent meals worked better than large ones. I kept ginger chews in my bag and sipped peppermint tea when the waves hit. Sometimes a cold smoothie helped settle things better than anything warm.

Constipation became a common and frustrating guest. Drinking more water and adding in prunes or gentle fiber-rich foods when I could tolerate them helped. I also relied on herbal teas and warm broths to gently nudge things along. Pain medications didn't make that any easier, so I learned to be proactive.

Mouth sores and dry mouth made food feel like sandpaper. I leaned into soft, soothing options like mashed potatoes, yogurt, applesauce, even pudding. Baking soda rinses (¼ tsp in 1 cup of water) became my go-to multiple times a day.

That awful metallic taste during chemo? Using plastic utensils helped more than I expected. Cold foods dulled the edge a bit, and citrus or mint occasionally cut through it. I carried lemon drops in my purse everywhere I went as well.

When I faced diarrhea, the BRAT diet of bananas, rice, applesauce, and toast, helped the most. I avoided caffeine, dairy, and anything greasy or spicy until things settled. Electrolyte drinks helped me stay hydrated and replaced what I was losing.

186

🍷 The Complicated Role of Alcohol

Let's just say it outright: I was a mess. I drank. More than I should have. Not to party. Not to celebrate. Not because I didn't know better. I drank to escape. I drank to avoid my fears and ignore my cheating husband. I drank to quiet the screaming voice in my head that kept asking, "What if this doesn't get better?" Sadly, alcohol let me step outside of the body that was falling apart. It blurred the edges of everything.

Hannah said it too. "I didn't drink much before cancer. But after the second round of chemo, I started having wine with dinner. Then wine *instead* of dinner. It helped me sleep. Helped me not feel. For a while, it worked. Until it didn't. I knew I was numbing. I just didn't know how else to keep going."

But here's what I didn't know. Or maybe I did and just didn't want to face it. Your liver is already doing overtime during chemo. That's where the drugs go to be processed. It's your internal detox station, and it's working full-time trying to filter out poison while keeping you alive. And there I was, pouring more work into it. I didn't think about that. I just thought about how I needed to feel nothing at all.

I started waking up with blood on my pillow. Nosebleeds that soaked the sheets. My gums bled every time I brushed my teeth. I bruised so easily it looked like I'd been in a bar fight I didn't remember. I chalked it up to chemo. And yes, that was part of it. But no one told me that alcohol can make all of that worse. No one said, "Hey, by the way, this might drop your platelet count even lower."

Looking back now, I can't tell you with certainty that alcohol caused any of that. But I can't tell you it didn't, either. And maybe more importantly, I can't ignore what it did to me emotionally. Alcohol became the thing I turned to instead of people. Instead of reaching out and saying, "I'm not okay," I poured another glass. It numbed the fears, but it numbed connection too. It created just enough distance between me and the people who might have helped me crawl out of that dark place. It made me quieter, lonelier, more withdrawn, and occasionally left me crying on the floor because communication seemed to be beyond my capabilities.

I told people I was doing fine. I wasn't.

Rachel shared something I think so many of us will understand. "Everyone kept saying how 'strong' I was. I clung to that. Smiled through the scans, joked through chemo, made memes and playlists and cookies. But at night, I fell apart. I avoided mirrors. I avoided silence. I avoided myself. Anything to not feel the grief."

So when I talk about alcohol now, it's not from a place of judgment. Believe me when. Say I'm not standing here wagging a finger at you. I'm standing here with the same alcohol-stained shame and wishing someone had handed me a truth I wasn't ready to hear back then. If you're drinking during cancer treatment, I get it. I really do. But I also want you to know this: your body is doing everything it can to keep you alive. If this is you, it's time to get help and give your body the best chance at healing.

That might mean skipping the wine. Not forever. Not as some grand declaration of self-denial. But just for now. Just long enough to let your liver breathe. Just long enough to stay a little clearer. Just long enough to feel instead of numb, and maybe reach out instead of pulling back.

And if you do decide to put down the glass, even just for today, I hope you can see that not as a punishment, but as a gift. A moment of mercy for your body. A little bit of kindness for your soul. Something that says, "I'm still here. I'm still fighting. And I want to stay."

Because you do. Even on the days when it's hard to say it out loud.

And you deserve to fight with every part of you, fully awake, fully present, and not alone.

And while we're being honest, I'll tell you this too: I was also a smoker.

Logically, you'd think a cancer diagnosis would've made me quit cold turkey. No point in giving myself *more* cancer, right? I know how it sounds from the outside. I see how it looks in black-and-white, especially to anyone who has never smoked or never stared down a life-threatening illness. But when I got that phone call, my first reaction wasn't to suddenly become the healthiest version of myself. It was to survive the next breath. I just needed to find a way to get through until it was all over.

And the truth is, I smoked more. Not because I didn't care. Not because I wanted to sabotage my healing. But because it was the only thing that made me feel like I had control over *anything* in that moment. It calmed my nerves when nothing else could. It gave me something to do with my hands while the rest of my world was crumbling. It was a coping tool. One that I knew wasn't good for me, but I wasn't aiming for "good." I was aiming for "bearable."

I'm not proud of it. But I'm also not ashamed anymore. Because I know now that I wasn't the only one. And if you're reading this and seeing yourself in it, if you're reaching for a cigarette or a drink or anything that makes the fear just a little quieter, I want you to know: you are not a failure. You are not weak. You are a human being going through something unimaginable.

No one teaches you how to navigate cancer *and* addiction *and* shame *and* grief all at once. But you are doing the best you can with what you've got. And if, at some point, you decide to make a different choice, if you decide to quit or to cut back or to reach for something else, I hope it comes from a place of love, not out of guilt or outside pressure.

Please know that you are worthy of love exactly as you are, and twice as much on your messiest days.

✔ Chapter Highlights

- Treatment often alters taste, appetite, and digestion, making eating difficult but still essential.

- Protect your favorite foods by not eating them during chemo to avoid lasting aversions.

- Nutrition during treatment supports healing, reduces side effects, and preserves strength.

- Side effects like nausea, mouth sores, metallic taste, and constipation can be eased through specific food choices and simple strategies.

- Staying hydrated helps flush out toxins, maintain energy, and manage symptoms.

- Alcohol can interfere with treatment, healing, and emotional well-being, especially when used to mask fear or stress.

- Gentle self-care through nutrition is a powerful act of love, not a punishment or a fix for the past.

💗 Key Takeaway

Nourishing your body during cancer isn't about guilt or blame. It's about honoring the version of you that is still here, still fighting, and still deserving of care, one sip, one bite, one breath at a time.

"I truly believe that everything happens for a reason."
—Giuliana Rancic; opened conversations on cancer and fertility preservation

16
Movement, Healing, and Letting People In

I didn't find healing through movement. Not at first. In fact, if you had asked me during treatment what role exercise played in my recovery, I probably would have laughed, or maybe maybe even cried. I was surviving, not sweating. Numbing out, not working out. My coping tools were alcohol, cigarettes and distraction, not yoga mats and sneakers. I was stuck in a toxic marriage, exhausted from chemo, and emotionally wrecked. The idea of taking a walk around the block felt about as possible as climbing Mount Everest in flip-flops. My body didn't feel like mine anymore, and I didn't trust it enough to move it.

But now, looking back, I can see what movement could have done for me. I don't mean in the punishing, gym-rat way we've all been guilted into thinking we need, but in a soul-soothing, breath-returning, "I still exist" kind of way. More about stretching the muscles, deep breaths and remembering who you are. Gentle movement can sometimes be the thing that starts to stitch you back together.

⊚ This Isn't About Fitness Goals

This chapter isn't here to lecture you about bouncing back, losing weight, hitting step counts, or posting gym selfies. This is chapter is helping you reconnect with your body after it's been through absolute hell. It's about honoring what's still working, even when so much feels broken. It's about breathing into tight spaces, stretching muscles that haven't moved in weeks, and taking small steps—not because you're chasing some external goal, but because you're learning to trust your body again.

Maybe that movement is lifting your arms over your head for the first time after surgery. Maybe it's walking to the mailbox. Maybe it's just sitting upright in bed and rolling your shoulders back because you've been curled in on yourself for days. That counts. Every little bit of movement is a quiet act of defiance against the heaviness that cancer brings.

You don't have to run marathons. And you don't need a color-coded fitness plan. You just need to move in a way that feels good to your body. That might be a few minutes of stretching while you wait for the kettle to boil. A walk around the backyard with your dog. A couple of deep breaths with your eyes closed. These aren't workouts, but a gentle reminder that your body, while changed, is still yours, and still worthy of care.

Moving After Surgery

When your body is fighting cancer, movement might be the last thing on your mind. It feels like a betrayal to even consider exercise when you're just trying to stay upright. But movement is one of the most healing things you can give yourself.

If you've had surgery, especially a mastectomy or lymph node removal, movement can feel terrifying. You don't want to break anything. You don't want to make it worse. But physical therapy exercises are often introduced early, not to push you, but to help you avoid complications like stiffness, loss of mobility, or lymphedema. The goal isn't to power through. It's to move gently. Slowly. One breath, one reach, one tiny stretch at a time.

Your arms might feel tight. Your chest might feel numb. You may be sore or scared. That's normal. But the more you begin to gently move, under the guidance of your care team, the more you start to remind your body that it's allowed to heal. That it doesn't have to stay frozen in pain.

Movement is just as much for your soul and your mindset as it is for your muscles. Walking through your neighborhood. Stretching in the living room. Doing gentle yoga, or putting on music and dancing like no one's watching, these are ways to lift the fog. To move the stuck energy. To reclaim just a little bit of control when everything else feels uncertain.

You don't need a gym membership and neon shorts. You just need a willingness to listen to your body and ask, "What do you need today?" And whatever the answer is, whether it's rest or a short walk or something in between, that's enough.

🌸 Start Small, Without Guilt

Let go of the pressure to "get back to normal." That old version of normal doesn't exist anymore. Recovery is a slow, steady reclaiming of the body you live in. Melanie D., who had DCIS surgery, once shared something that stuck with me. She said, "I remember how walking even a short distance left me winded after surgery. But I promised myself I'd walk to the end of the driveway every morning. It wasn't much, but it made me feel like I had some say in my recovery. Eventually I could make it around the block. And then a little further. I wasn't chasing a goal, I was reclaiming my life one breath at a time."

There is no gold medal waiting for you at the end of this. If your big win today is getting out of bed and walking to the mailbox, then you've already succeeded. You're not in competition with anyone, not even the version of yourself from before.

Movement doesn't have to be structured or sweaty. It can be lying on the floor with your legs up the wall, doing slow circles with your arms, or wiggling your toes to a song that makes you feel alive again. It invites you to go slow, listen carefully, and savor the miracle of being in your body, even if that body feels foreign right now. There's no rush. Just move when it feels right, and let that be enough.

So, if you're feeling up for it, start small. Chair yoga, gentle tai chi, or just wiggling in your seat to a favorite song. Every little movement counts. And on the days when all you manage is rolling out of bed and brushing your teeth? That counts too. You're showing up. You're trying. Celebrate that.

💤 What Real Self-Care Looks Like

Let's get one thing straight. Real self-care isn't bubble baths and bath bombs, unless that's what you need (and if it is, go soak like the goddess you are). Sometimes, self-care looks like sleeping in without guilt because your body is healing on a cellular level. It looks like wearing the softest pajamas you own all day long because every seam feels like sandpaper. It's skipping the phone calls and muting the group chat because silence feels kinder than conversation.

Carmen said it perfectly: "Self-care used to mean bubble baths and massages. But during treatment, it meant asking for help. Saying no. Taking naps in the middle of the day and not feeling guilty about it. It meant letting people love me even when I didn't feel lovable."

Real self-care might mean letting your best friend clean your kitchen, even when you cringe at the thought of someone seeing your sink full of dishes. It's crying into your dog's fur or rewatching the dumbest comedy for the third time this week just because it makes you laugh. It's canceling plans without apology, ordering takeout three nights in a row, and trusting that the people who love you will understand.

Melissa shared, "I was always the doer. The fixer. The one who handled everything. Cancer made me stop. It forced me to rest. And I had to learn to stop seeing rest as weakness."

Tasha told me, "Every night after treatment, I'd light a candle and sit in silence. Five minutes, no phone, no noise. It was my way of saying, 'You made it through another day.' That small ritual saved me more times than I can count."

Self-care during cancer is rarely glamorous. It's gritty. Tender. Awkward. Honest. And yours might not look like anyone else's. But that's okay. It's not for anyone else. It's for you.

Energy Conservation Isn't Failure

Here's your permission slip: you don't need to do everything. Not now. Not even close. You're not falling short by needing rest, you're making the wise choice to survive with what little energy you have. Sit while folding laundry. Use the damn shower chair. Let grocery delivery save you a trip. Choose two things that actually matter today, and let the rest fall away without guilt.

You're in the middle of a physical and emotional crisis, and it's taking every ounce of strength you have to keep going. Don't waste your energy trying to meet some invisible standard. You're not here to impress anyone. You're here to heal.

And if healing looks like a nap, a microwaved meal, and doing absolutely nothing else that day, then you're doing it right.

❀ Finding Peace in Quiet Things

When the noise gets too loud and the overwhelm becomes too much, give yourself permission to disappear into something quiet. Color outside the lines. Knit a row, unravel it, knit it again. Tend to a stubborn little plant that just won't die. Work on a puzzle with no edge pieces. Play a ridiculous game on your phone. Dance around your kitchen in fuzzy socks with a wooden spoon as your mic. Write a letter you'll never send, just to get the thoughts out.

And if you ever find yourself with a little extra energy, or just need to shift focus, consider putting together a small care kit for someone else going through treatment. A cozy pair of socks, a journal, a few mints, a gentle lotion. Something simple. Sometimes, helping someone else reminds you that you're not alone either. That there's a strange kind of peace in shared struggle.

What matters most isn't the size of your effort. It's that you keep choosing moments of calm, even when everything around you feels like chaos. Those five quiet minutes matter. They're medicine.

❀ Self-Care Means Letting People In

We often think of self-care as the picture-perfect stuff like bubble baths, candles, breathing exercises. But when you're deep in the thick of it, self-care is so much messier and so much more essential. It's more like a series of small, deliberate choices that help you not completely unravel. Reminding yourself again and again that your value isn't tied to how productive or helpful you are. Right now, healing is your only job, and that job is sacred.

Still, letting go can feel impossible. Especially for those of us who've made a habit of doing everything for everyone. Many of us were raised to be caretakers. We know how to anticipate needs, how to smooth over the hard parts, how to take care of people even when we're running on empty. We are maternal, even if we aren't mothers. So when it's our turn to be the one in need, we freeze. It feels foreign. Like failure or some kind of weakness.

Jess admitted, "I've always been the helper, not the one who needs help. But cancer flipped that. I had to learn how to receive without

195

apologizing. The first time someone brought dinner, I cried in the bathroom. Not because I was embarrassed, but because I felt so loved, and I didn't know how to process that."

But needing help doesn't mean you're broken. You could just use some assistance, in whatever way that might look for you.

Letting someone fold your laundry or bring you soup or just sit next to you in silence isn't giving up your independence. You're choosing connection, and letting love in. And love, especially the kind that shows up with casseroles and clean socks, is one of the strongest healing agents we have.

Denise shared, "It took me a long time to accept rides to appointments or say yes when someone offered to clean my house. I kept thinking, 'I don't want to be a burden.' But I was exhausted. And when I finally let people help, I realized they *wanted* to. It made them feel useful. It connected us."

So please, don't close the door on help. Crack it open. Let someone in. Let them remind you that you're not alone.

▨ You're Still in Charge

Asking for help can feel like giving up control, and let's be honest—sometimes the way people help makes you want to scream into a pillow. Maybe you like the dishwasher loaded a certain way. Maybe the sight of someone else folding your towels wrong makes your skin crawl. That's okay. Accepting help doesn't mean surrendering all your standards or giving up on what matters to you.

Think of it like this: You're still the captain of this ship. Sure, you're not mopping the deck or hoisting the sails right now, but you're steering. You get to call the plays. You decide what needs doing, when, and by whom. If someone offers to cook dinner, you can still pick the recipe, or veto the one you know nobody eats. If someone wants to tidy the house, make a list. Be as specific or as vague as you need to be. And if you need uninterrupted rest, schedule it in. Put it on the sacred team calendar and let them know nap time is non-negotiable. You're still in charge, just in a different way.

🔑 Breaking the Silent Standoff

Let's talk about your circle of people: your friends, coworkers, neighbors, even the random acquaintance who said, "Let me know if you need anything." The thing is, most of them genuinely want to help. They just don't know how. They're afraid of being intrusive, saying the wrong thing, or stepping on your already-frayed nerves. So when you say "I'm fine," they believe you. They back away, not because they don't care, but because they think they're honoring your space. They're trying to be respectful.

So while you're sitting there, barely holding it together, wishing someone would just show up with soup or scrub your bathroom, think about how "I'm fine" isn't the answer you want to give. But since you never asked, they never came. Welcome to the world's most frustrating silent standoff.

Here's how we break it: with words. I know, I know. Vulnerability isn't always easy. But saying something is better than leaving everyone guessing. Try, "I'm not okay, but I don't know what help looks like yet." Or, "I need support, but I'm not great at asking." You don't need a formal speech. You just need to crack open the door so people know they're welcome inside.

🩶 Let People Love You

And then there are the ones who already know how to show up. The quiet heroes who don't wait for permission. Kathy, one of the women I spoke with, told me about her daughter who flew in during treatment and cleaned her entire kitchen while she slept. No fanfare. No asking. No hesitation. "She knew I wouldn't say yes, so she just showed up anyway," Kathy told me, blinking back tears. "That moment taught me that love sometimes looks like doing the thing no one asked for."

Kendra experienced that same quiet care in her neighborhood. "I remember my neighbor leaving a pot of soup on the porch with a sticky note that said, 'No need to talk, just soup.' It was everything. Some days, the quietest kindness was the loudest comfort."

Here's a secret though: people do want to help. They need something to do. It doesn't need to be a grand gesture, but something small, specific, and doable can give them a way in. Ask for a Monday morning text, a store run for toothpaste and Gatorade, a walk for the dog once a week.

Tiny things. Tangible things. Things that make life just a little easier for you, and little lighter for them. You are giving people a way to show up and be part of your healing, even if they can't fix a damn thing.

You are not a burden. You are not too much. And you are absolutely not failing. No matter what your mind is saying.

You are walking through something enormous. And you are encouraged to accept backup.

Let them come. Let them carry something, even if it's small. Let yourself be held. Because you don't have to do this alone.

And more importantly, you were never supposed to.

Joyce Let Them Love Her

Joyce didn't ask for help, but she didn't turn it away either. And because of that, she experienced what it truly means to be surrounded by grace.

Her teenage children didn't complain. They didn't crumble. They did what needed to be done, quietly and with more strength than most adults. Her husband stood beside her with calm reassurance, supporting every decision she made. His steady presence helped carry her through even the hardest days.

But what really surprised her was how her newer connections in the teachers and staff at her job, rallied for her like lifelong friends. They helped her stay on top of things at work. They wrapped and delivered Christmas presents for her kids. They showed up, not because they had to, but because they wanted to.

Her church family, too, was relentless in their love. Meals. Cards. Prayers. Envelopes with enough money for the long drives to Houston showing up at just the right time.

Joyce didn't fight their kindness. She let it in. She let people love her, and in doing so, she gave them the chance to be part of her healing.

✔ Chapter Highlights

- Movement during and after treatment can support healing, both physically and emotionally.

- Gentle, non-demanding exercises (like walking, stretching, or chair yoga) help ease symptoms and reconnect you with your body.

- Energy conservation is essential. Doing less is not failure, it's wisdom.

- Self-care is not selfish or indulgent; it's a survival strategy.

- Asking for help doesn't mean giving up control, it means building a support system that works for you.

- Clear communication allows loved ones to show up in meaningful ways.

♡ Key Takeaway

Healing is about giving yourself permission to receive care from others, as much as you give it.

"I had both breasts removed because now I have zero chance of having breast cancer."
—*Wanda Sykes; discussed preventive mastectomy after DCIS diagnosis*

17
After the Applause: What Comes Next

When treatment ends, people expect you to celebrate. "You made it!" they say, their voices bright with relief and expectation. But for many of us, the hardest part begins when the fight is over.

Survivorship wasn't a victory parade for me. It was just another step in my struggle. My body was still aching, my emotions frayed, and what remained of my life, was scattered in pieces I couldn't carry. I was navigating a bitter divorce, forced to leave my home with nothing but my Jeep, a few changes of clothes, and my dog. My children stayed behind with my ex because, at the time, I had no way to provide the stability my girls deserved. That decision still aches in the deepest parts of me, but I know it was the right one at the time, given the impossible choices in front of me.

When I told my husband I wanted a divorce after discovering his affairs, he retaliated in ways I wasn't prepared for. He cut off my access to our joint bank accounts and left me financially paralyzed. He had been the primary earner. I couldn't afford a lawyer. The court system didn't recognize my years of military service, or the fact that I had given up my career to raise our kids and support his career. It didn't matter that I had adopted his daughter and loved her like my own for the past 10 years. In the end, he was granted full custody. I received no alimony, no part of his military retirement, and was ordered to pay him $500 a month in child support.

He kept the house. The valuables. And even my personal belongings, including things like my motorcycle helmet, my leather chaps, my photo albums filled with memories from my childhood and my time in the Navy. Years later, he gave back a few of the things he no longer wanted, passing them through our daughter like hand-me-downs from a life I wasn't allowed to keep. And when I asked why he was treating me like that, when I tried to plead for fairness or even an ounce of decency, he gaslit me. Twisted every conversation. Turned it all around until I started questioning my own memory of events, wondering if maybe I was the problem after all.

For a while, I lived out of my Jeep, surviving on snacks from gas stations and adrenaline. I picked up second jobs, but the income was eaten up by wage garnishments before I could even hold the check in my hand. I couldn't catch a break. I was tired. Hungry. Embarrassed. My mother sent me just enough to rent a small apartment, but that didn't last long. Rent and child support couldn't coexist. Eventually, I packed what little I had and moved to Georgia to live with friends. It wasn't where I imagined life taking me, but it was all I had left.

And oddly enough, that's where real healing began. Survivorship isn't just about hearing the words "No Evidence of Disease." It's not only a clean scan or an end date on the calendar. Survivorship is about learning to live again. Learning how to move forward, not just because you made it through, but because you've decided you're worth it, fully, and on your own terms.

I wasn't just recovering from cancer. I was healing from betrayal, from abandonment, from the violent unraveling of everything I thought I could count on. That kind of trauma doesn't just wash away with time. It soaks into your bones. It whispers when you're quiet. It took years before I could even begin writing this book. But I'm here now, not because everything is magically okay, but because therapy, time, and genuine love created enough space for reflection.

It took me nine years to marry again. And this time, I chose a different kind of man. He doesn't try to fix everything. He doesn't feel the need to control or rescue me. He just shows up, fully, with quiet strength and patience. He stands beside me, not over me. He supports me, listens to me, and is a partner in life. That simple, steady presence gave me something I hadn't felt in years: safety.

The Good That Follows

It would be easy to stop the story at the heartbreak, the loss, the chaos that came after cancer. But that wouldn't be the full truth. Because while some people left, others showed up. And their presence, quiet and consistent, mattered more than they probably know.

Some of them were strangers at first. A friend of a friend who offered a room when I had nowhere to go. A coworker who packed an extra sandwich each day without ever making a big deal out of it. A boss that let me bring my daughter to work on days she didn't have school, rather than miss spending time with her. Kindness came in small, scattered doses. Not all at once, not neatly packaged, but in a way that slowly stitched me back together. I took whatever I could get in those days, and I really feel like those little gestures helped me survive.

Healing didn't arrive as some grand, shining moment. It came in slivers. A deep breath that didn't come with panic. A laugh that didn't carry guilt. A morning when I woke up and didn't immediately feel dread. It was letting go of the burdens I never should've carried in the first place, and beginning to build a life that felt like mine.

Joyce's story reminded me that healing doesn't look the same for everyone. Her journey wasn't wrapped in divorce or betrayal, but it still had its pain. And yet, she was held by her family, her friends, and her church. She let people in, let them carry her when she couldn't walk on her own. There was something incredibly brave about the way she received love. She didn't wear strength like armor. For her, it was all grace.

🔄 The Silent Second Battle

When the chemo stops dripping and the radiation machine powers down, people tend to exhale. They throw around words like "survivor" and "strong" and "You did it!" And they mean well. But while they celebrate, you're left standing in the aftermath. The noise dies down. The appointments stop. The help and support fades away. The calendar that once dictated your every move suddenly becomes a blank slate. And that blankness can be terrifying.

During treatment, you have structure. You have doctors, nurses, a plan, a path. But once it's all done, the scaffolding vanishes. And you're left with nothing but the echoes of what you've been through. The world expects you to bounce back, to return to the version of you they remember. But that version doesn't exist anymore. Something big inside you has changed. You feel things differently now. You see life as raw, fragile, and beautifully complicated. And yet, the world keeps spinning like nothing ever happened. You feel invisible.

During my divorce, I was still technically in treatment. Homeless while finishing my radiation treatments. Hanging out in parks to let my children play for a few hours before handing them back and returning to my car for the night. I smiled through it for them, but my soul felt like it was unraveling. And while I was in survival mode, my closest friend was falling apart too. Her marriage had ended, and she was devastated. But I wasn't there for her. I didn't call. I didn't even know. Not because I didn't care, but because I was barely holding my own head above water. It was like I was living in a bubble, just trying to survive from day to day.

Our friendship didn't survive that silence. We tried to patch it over the years, but the wound was too deep, and the timing was never quite right. She never understood and never stopped being angry with me. I still wonder, what if I had made just one phone call? Would things have turned out differently? Maybe. Maybe not. But that's what trauma does. It distorts time. It blurs your ability to show up. It makes you forget how to reach out, even when your heart is breaking for someone else.

The truth is, I didn't have the capacity to be there for her. I barely had enough to be there for myself. And I've had to learn to forgive myself for that.

Because the aftermath of cancer isn't just physical. It's emotional. It's relational. It's the quiet collapse that happens after the world assumes you're okay.

Healing isn't a finish line. It's a slow return to yourself, with plenty of detours, missteps, and lessons along the way.

And if all you've done today is keep breathing, that's enough. Keep it up you're doing just fine.

The Emotional Landscape of Survivorship

Survivorship stirs up a storm of emotions no one prepares you for. It can feel like being dropped into unfamiliar territory with no map and no instructions.

There's guilt for surviving when others didn't, for not feeling more grateful, for struggling when you're "supposed" to feel lucky.

There's fear that lurks in every ache or strange twinge, a fear that maybe the cancer is back, that maybe your body will betray you again.

There's grief, deep and aching, for the person you were before, for the things you lost, for the time that slipped through your fingers during treatment.

And then, out of nowhere, there are bursts of joy in the strangest, most beautiful moments. Moments of bliss when the sun hits your skin just right, or you laugh so hard you forget, for a second, what you've been through.

There's anger too. Anger at the unfairness of it all. At the broken systems. At your own body. At the way some people disappear when you need them most.

And beneath it all, there's loneliness. The kind of loneliness that settles in when the world thinks you're "better," but you're still trying to find your footing in a life that looks familiar but feels completely different.

This part of the journey is as personal as it is unpredictable. Some days, you feel like you're soaring, unshakable in your strength. Other days, you're just trying to crawl through the ashes of everything that changed. And the truth is, all of it counts. Every feeling. Every setback. Every small victory. This is survivorship. And you're allowed to feel every messy, complicated piece of it. Most of all, you're allowed to grow and heal at your own pace.

Melissa W., Diagnosed at 38

My diagnosis came through MyChart on a quiet Saturday evening. Stage zero DCIS. Early and treatable, they said. But it didn't feel like good news. It felt like the ground cracked beneath me. I was shaking. Terrified.

A call from Dr. MJ, a dear friend and physician, was the rope I clung to. Her calm voice walked me through what I couldn't yet comprehend. I'd been through so much in my life: depression, PTSD, unimaginable loss. But suddenly, I saw something I hadn't seen in years: choice. I could choose my path. I chose a double mastectomy.

Surgery was scheduled for September 8. It was the anniversary of my late fiancé's death. At first, I resisted. But then I realized maybe he was guiding me. I cried walking in, and my mother broke down beside me. The nurse who held my hand said, "You are so strong to be here."

Post-op, the pathology confirmed it: more cancer was forming. My decision had been more than brave. It had also been a wise choice. And in the days that followed, something shifted. I felt lighter. Somehow, more like myself.

To mark the one-year anniversary of my mastectomy, I got a tattoo across my chest. A piece of art over the place where trauma had once lived. I was claiming my story. These scars became part of the masterpiece of my life.

I started over. Left a job that didn't see me. Stopped apologizing. Started loving myself. Survivorship didn't erase the guilt. It deepened my empathy. I use my voice to hold space for others still in the dark.

Cancer didn't destroy me. It opened me up.

Thriving, Not Just Surviving

Being a survivor might feel like the final chapter, but don't look at it that way. Instead, it's the doorway to the next part of your life.

Thriving means living your life with purpose. Learning to reclaim joy. Laughing without apology. Saying yes to what feeds you and no to what drains you. It's about choosing life in small, sacred ways.

Cancer taught me to stop postponing happiness. To stop waiting for the perfect moment to celebrate. The moment is now. Wear the outfit. Take the trip. Eat the dessert. Say the words. Take the picture.

To every woman still dreaming, healing, and building: I see you. I honor you. You are not broken. You are becoming the greater, freer version of yourself.

✒ Gerry W. K., Diagnosed at 60

At 60, I was used to mammograms. My breasts had been cystic since my twenties. But one scan revealed something new. Suspicious calcifications. A biopsy. Then the call: DCIS. And after surgery? Invasive ductal carcinoma. Stage 1. Chemo and radiation.

At the same time, I was caring for my mother, who was dying of kidney failure. I tried to shield her from my diagnosis, and wore a brave face. She passed away between my chemo and radiation. It gutted me.

But amid the sorrow came joy. Two grandbabies were born. My five-year-old granddaughter looked at my bald head and said, "You look beautiful." She offered me her Tinkerbell tiara. That tiny act held so much love for me.

Cancer didn't strip everything away for me. It uncovered strength I didn't know I had. I began exercising, gained energy, lost weight. Not because of illness, but because I wanted to live my life differently.

My cousin, also diagnosed, became my anchor. We called ourselves the "chemo-sabes." We laughed and cried through it all. I stopped all meds after two years. She powered through. Both of us honored our own paths.

I now volunteer with Living Beyond Breast Cancer. I answer calls from newly diagnosed women. I let them know: it's scary, but you'll get through. I write poetry, including a piece called "Scars." Because healing might be messy, but it's real.

Cancer changed me. It both softened and strengthened me. I remember my mother. I wear my granddaughter's love like a crown. And I move forward, scarred, but whole.

🔥 Becoming the Phoenix

Cancer didn't just take things from you. It burned your life down to the bones. It stripped away the noise, the distractions, the illusions. And what was left in the rubble was raw, painful, and unrecognizable. But as any gardener can tell you, ashes make good soil. From that devastation, something new begins.

207

You are not the same person you were before. You carry a deeper wisdom now. A softness that doesn't equal weakness. A bravery born from surviving the unthinkable. You feel more. You notice more. You protect your peace like a sacred thing. You listen to your intuition, because it has earned your trust.

Now is the time to build the life you want, not the one you settled for before. This is your opportunity to plant new dreams, even if they're small and shaky at first. Say no to what drains you. Say yes to what sets your soul on fire. Take up space. Let your presence be loud or quiet, bold or tender, but let it be yours.

You have earned every step of this new becoming. Through fire and wreckage, you found a way to rise. And what you are now is someone fierce. Someone free. Someone who knows exactly how much it costs to survive, and chooses to live fully anyway.

Chrissy: Still Standing, Still Smiling, and Always Choosing Joy

My name is Chrissy, and after 4 ½ years of chemotherapy, radiation, and three surgeries, including a double mastectomy, I am officially in remission. And wow, what a ride it's been.

It all started in April of 2019, when I was dealing with what I thought was a pesky sinus infection. I went to the doctor, got some antibiotics, and figured it would clear up. Around the same time, I found a lump in my left armpit during a self-breast exam. I even had my husband, Eric, double-check. We both thought it might be nothing, but I kept an eye on it.

Over the next few months, I was back and forth to the doctor. Sinus infections. Earaches. Sore throats. I even joked that I had developed a "third boob" in my armpit. I was constantly tired, but chalked it up to working too much. And since I'd just turned 50 that October, I figured maybe this was what midlife felt like. (Can I go back to 49, please?)

By November, I wasn't just tired, I was bone tired! So I went back to the doctor, who finally took things seriously. He ordered bloodwork and scans. A day later, I got a call. Something was definitely off. The CA-125 levels were high, and they suspected lymphoma. Within days, I had a port placed and a biopsy scheduled. Things were moving so fast I barely had time to think, let alone process the words *cancer patient*, but that's exactly what I had become.

On December 11, Eric and I sat in stunned silence as the surgeon told us my biopsy was "inconclusive" but likely metastatic cancer, possibly from the breast. Or possibly not. In other words, no one knew where it was coming from. That punch-in-the-gut moment? Yep. There it was.

More appointments, more waiting, more uncertainty. Until finally, on Christmas Eve, my oncologist called. She apologized for calling on the holiday but said she couldn't wait. The biopsy review from the Cleveland Clinic had come in. It was breast cancer. Triple Negative. Stage 3C. And you know what? I was relieved. *Relieved*. At least now we knew what we were dealing with. The not-knowing had been worse than the diagnosis.

That Christmas was one I'll never forget. I remember watching my adult kids open gifts, soaking in every smile, every laugh, every yawn. I couldn't bear the thought of missing weddings or grandbabies or even another Christmas morning. And that's when it hit me. I was not going down without a fight.

Chemo started January 6. I shaved my head on January 9, because if cancer was going to take my hair, I'd be the one to hand it over. I even had a mantra: **Choose Joy**. I wore it on my shirts. My friends and family wore it too, especially on chemo days. It became more than just a slogan. It was a mindset. A reminder that no matter how brutal the treatment was, cancer wasn't allowed to steal my joy.

And let me tell you, chemo *was* brutal. The Red Devil lived up to its name, and I had an allergic reaction to Taxol. I worked from home during treatment, which sounds easier than it was. I was tired. My bones ached. I couldn't sleep. But I pushed through. I refused to let cancer take the driver's seat.

Then came the double mastectomy in June 2020. I was at peace with it. My boobs had served their purpose, and quite frankly, they had turned against me. What I wasn't at peace with was the surgeon's handiwork. Let's just say it looked like he was blindfolded. Thankfully, my oncologist referred me to someone who knew what they were doing, and I had a corrective surgery in September.

Radiation came next. And let me tell you, if I had to choose between chemo and radiation? I'd take chemo. Hands down. Radiation was no joke. Burns, mouth sores, a throat that felt like I'd swallowed sandpaper. I couldn't eat. I was constantly dehydrated. But somehow, I got through it.

And then, just when I thought I could breathe, a new lump showed up. I was placed on Xeloda, an oral chemo drug that nearly killed me. Four weeks in the hospital later, I found myself angry. Frustrated. Tired of this fight. But then I heard my own voice whispering, *Choose Joy*. Ugh. I hate when I'm right.

Cancer isn't just the appointments, the pills, the scars. It's also the moments in between, the ones that keep you going. My kids knew how scared I was, so they created "Flamingo Fridays." Every week, they gave me a flamingo-themed surprise: rubber flamingos hidden around the house, silly gifts from Amazon. It gave us all something to smile about.

I've had some memorable moments post-mastectomy too. Like the time I tried wearing knitted knockers in my swimsuit and one popped out in the pool. Yep. Had to swim after it like I was on a rescue mission. Now I just rock the flat look. When we go out to our local pub and Eric orders the "busty breasts" off the menu, I always chime in with, "Of course he wants two, that's the only kind he gets!" Watching the waitstaff try to figure out how to respond is one of my favorite pastimes.

But underneath the laughter is the truth. This journey changed me. I walk with a cane now because of neuropathy in my feet. I can't drive. I can't work. I lost a lot of independence. I deal with lymphedema and chronic fatigue. The weight gain, hair changes, and scars sometimes make me feel like a stranger in my own body. I've had to grieve the old me. I've had to fight to find who I am now.

But I'm getting there. I'm in therapy. I'm learning how to dress this new body. I'm reconnecting with myself. Some days are hard. Some days, I still cry. But most days, I laugh. I sit in my happy place surrounded by flowers, listening to the birds sing, and I remember that I'm still here. I'm beating the odds. And I'll never stop choosing joy.

Cancer didn't get the last word, I did.

✅ Chapter Highlights

- Survivorship doesn't always feel like a celebration. It can be the beginning of a new, lonely, and overwhelming chapter.

- The emotional weight of survivorship includes fear, grief, guilt, and the difficult process of rebuilding identity and relationships.

- Friendship and connection can be reshaped, or lost, by trauma, even when both people are doing their best.

- Thriving doesn't mean "bouncing back." It means living with intention, honoring your growth, and reclaiming your joy.

- Cancer may have burned everything down, but you get to choose what rises from the ashes.

💜 Key Takeaway

Life after cancer isn't about returning to who you were—it's about honoring who you've become. Thriving means making room for joy, for grief, for healing, and for becoming whole in a brand new way.

"Just when the caterpillar thought the world was over, it became a butterfly."
—Proverb

18
The Mountain Lion in the Fridge: Life After Cancer

After treatment ended and the dust began to settle, I was hit with something no one had warned me about: a form of PTSD. The debilitating fear of recurrence. It wasn't loud. It didn't come crashing in. It was quieter than that, more subtle. A dull hum in the background of every day. Every tiny ache or odd sensation became a red flag. A twinge in my side? Cancer. A bruise I couldn't explain? Obviously cancer. A headache? Cancer, of course. I couldn't tell if I was being paranoid or just more aware, but I lived in a heightened state of attention, constantly scanning my body for signs of betrayal for years afterwards.

And that fear still continues to follow me into every appointment, every scan, every blood test. Even seventeen years later, I still cry every time I get a mammogram. The smell of the antiseptic wipes, the cold of the machine, the waiting room chatter. It all triggers that same tightness in my chest. I tremble and hold my breath, fighting the wave of panic that rises as the plates press down, just praying to make it through the appointment. I tell myself to stay still, to breathe, to be brave. But by the time it's over, the tears have started to come anyway. I rush to the tiny changing room, desperate to escape, to hide, to let the fear leak out in private. Because no matter how many years have passed, part of me is still that terrified woman waiting for someone to say the words that will change everything again.

And then, just to add another layer of anxiety, I no longer had health insurance after my divorce. Being a veteran, I transitioned over to the VA for follow-up care, and I'll be honest, my stomach dropped at the thought. The VA doesn't exactly have a stellar reputation when it comes to women's health, and I wasn't sure I'd be taken seriously. But to my surprise, the VA in Atlanta proved me wrong in all the best ways. They wrapped their arms around me with care and consistency. They scheduled diagnostic mammograms, ultrasounds, MRIs. Every three months, I was in their office. And for the first time in a long time, I felt watched over. Protected and safe.

Eventually, those checkups spaced out. Every six months. Then once a year. These days, I go annually for a diagnostic mammogram. And if anything looks off, they follow up right away with an ultrasound. No delay, no guessing. At my most recent mammogram, however, my doctor had asked for a diagnostic mammogram, as she always has, and the woman that did the mammogram took it upon herself to change it to a regular instead of diagnostic. That meant that I had to wait a week or more to get my results, because she didn't want to have the radiologist look at the results that same day while I was there. I was very angry about that, especially since I knew my doctor had requested the diagnostic. Unfortunately, people that have never experienced cancer don't understand that even after 17 years, you can still be affected by past experiences. Waiting was not okay with me, and it if it's not something you're able to face, then you shouldn't have to. Talk with your doctor about diagnostic mammograms, and don't be afraid to speak up if someone tries to change it.

💔 Rebuilding After Loss

In the beginning, I carried anger like a second skin. Anger at cancer. At God. At my ex-husband. At losing custody of my children. At being homeless. At friends who disappeared when things got too messy. I was furious at the way life had unraveled, thread by thread, until I didn't recognize the fabric of it anymore. But over the years, as my life slowly started to come back together, something softer started to grow in its place. I found joy in spending time with my children. I laughed again. I breathed easier. And eventually, I started to build a new life from the ashes of the old one.

Nine years after my divorce, I remarried.

And after everything, I never thought I would even want to find love again. I had been so hurt, by betrayal, by abandonment, by the lies, that I couldn't imagine letting anyone close to me again. When I met my now-husband, I wasn't looking for love. I wasn't even looking for a relationship. But he didn't push. He didn't try to fix me or chase me. He just stood there, patient, calm, steady, and let me come to him when I was ready. It took four years before he proposed. Four years of rebuilding trust, of relearning what love could look like, of slowly loosening the armor I had worn for far too long.

I won't like, we fought. A lot. And it was mostly my fault. I was overly defensive and tended to jump to conclusions when things got hard. He had to constantly remind me that he's not my ex husband. I couldn't treat him like he did something wrong, unless he actually did something wrong! This was *really* hard for me, but he was so patient with me.

When we finally got married, it wasn't flashy or loud. It was quiet. Intentional. Surrounded by our children and only the closest friends and family. It was a powerful moment of choosing each other, not because we needed to, but because we wanted to. It was the first time in a long time that I believed in love again. Not just the love between two people, but the kind of love that lets you see yourself clearly and still offers grace. His love didn't demand anything from me. It created space for me to grow, to heal, and to finally see myself as worthy again.

Now, when I look back on everything I went through, the cancer, the divorce, the loss, the grief, it doesn't sting the way it used to. The pain is still part of the story, but it no longer holds the pen. I've made peace with it all. And it took years, but it was worth every step.

✎ What I Wish I'd Known

These days, I feel this deep compulsion to help others. Not because I have it all figured out, but because I remember how dark and confusing those days were when I didn't know where to turn. I feel a pull to open up the old scars. To speak out loud the parts most people keep hidden. Not for sympathy, and definitely not for shock value. But because I truly believe that sharing what I went through, especially the parts my story that I wish I could rewrite, might help someone else avoid falling into the same holes I did.

My story isn't just about how hard cancer was. It's a reflection on what happens when you try to carry too much, for too long, in silence. It's about what gets lost when you ignore your own emotional needs, when you smile through pain, when you wait too long to say, "I need help." If I could go back, I would have reached out sooner. I would have let people in. I would have admitted, even just to myself, that I was drowning.

So if you're in the thick of it right now, if you're hurting, unsure, scared about what comes next, please hear me: peace is possible. Healing is possible. And real love, the gentle kind, the patient kind, the kind that grows with you, is still possible too.

And if sharing the messy, ugly, vulnerable parts of my journey helps light even one small corner of the path for someone else, then every scar I've reopened to write this book has been worth it. Every single one.

⚠ Alicia's Story: Quiet Panic and Private Pain

Alicia had triple-negative breast cancer, one of the most aggressive forms, and beat it after six months of intense chemo and a double mastectomy. On the outside, she looked like the poster child for survival: brave, bald, smiling through treatment. But privately, she was unraveling. "I didn't tell anyone how scared I was," she said. "Everyone wanted me to be strong, so I played the part."

Even after treatment ended, she couldn't shake the sense that something bad was around the corner. Every cold, every bruise, every ache sent her spiraling. It wasn't until she found an online forum filled with other women whispering the same thoughts—*What if it's back? Am I crazy? Why can't I relax?*—that she realized she wasn't alone. Just knowing that others had those same midnight fears helped her feel more grounded. She still worries sometimes, but now she knows how to talk herself down, and who to call when she can't.

😨 More Than Anxiety: PTSD After Cancer

For many of us, the fear of recurrence isn't just anxiety, it's real trauma. The body remembers what the mind tries to forget. One faint chemical scent, the beeping of a monitor, the sharp sting of antiseptic in the air, even the sound of Velcro on a blood pressure cuff can yank you straight back into the chemo room without warning. You might be years out from treatment. Your labs might be perfect. But your stomach still twists, your heart still races, and suddenly, it's infusion day all over again.

That's not in your head. That's post-traumatic stress.

PTSD after cancer doesn't always look the way people expect. It doesn't always announce itself with flashbacks or nightmares. Sometimes it hides in the little things, irritability that seems to come from nowhere, trouble sleeping, or an inexplicable wave of tears while folding towels. You might notice it creeping in around scan time, that quiet dread pooling in your chest. You can't focus. Your fuse is shorter. Your thoughts are already playing out worst-case scenarios, even if you're smiling on the outside.

One survivor told me that every time a checkup approached, she found herself snapping at her kids, lashing out over tiny things. She didn't feel scared, not consciously. But her body knew. Her nervous system had already hit the panic button. It wasn't until a therapist gently named it, "This might be PTSD," that she finally let herself cry. It wasn't drama. It was a nervous system begging for safety.

You don't have to "push through" it. You don't have to pretend you're fine.

There are trauma-informed therapists who understand the unique weight cancer survivors carry. There are support groups where you don't have to explain what it feels like to live with a mountain lion pacing in your chest. And there are grounding tools—deep breaths, warm tea, walking barefoot in the grass—that help bring your body back to the present moment, where you are safe.

You are not weak for feeling this way. You are strong—for surviving something terrifying, for continuing to show up, and for being willing to name the truth of what you carry.

Naming it is how we begin to heal.

🐾 The Mountain Lion in the Fridge

There's a story that gets passed around the breast cancer community. One that somehow captures the bizarre, relentless, surreal nature of what survivorship can feel like. It's called *the mountain lion in the fridge*. And once you hear it, you never forget it.

It goes like this: One day, you open your refrigerator, and there's a mountain lion inside. No one can explain why it's there. All you know is that it's trying to kill you. Your only shot at survival? Run up a mountain to find a bear. A literal bear. So you run. The mountain lion chases you. Your friends want to help, but they can't fight this thing for you. They stand on the sidelines shouting encouragement, tossing orange slices and water bottles your way, doing what they can, but the climb itself is yours alone.

At some point, someone you love jumps in to help. They mean well, but they get hurt too. Maybe not the same way, but the impact is real. You keep running. You're bleeding and bruised. Eventually, by some wild stroke of timing, or medicine, or both, you find the bear. The bear fights the mountain lion. It wins, but not before the lion mauls you again. Because nothing about this has been clean or fair or simple.

When it's all over, people cheer. They call you brave. They tell you how inspiring you are. They bring cake and balloons. You get to ring a bell to celebrate. But inside, you're exhausted. Limping and still bleeding. Your body and spirit are barely held together with duct tape, zip ties and hope.

And all anyone says is, "Aren't you glad it's over?"

Meanwhile, you're standing there thinking, "I never wanted to climb this mountain in the first place, and now I'm afraid every time I open my fridge."

That's what fear of recurrence feels like. The mountain lion may be gone, but you never forget that it was real. That it was in your fridge, and that it could come back. So even when you're smiling, grocery shopping, booking vacations, doing all the "normal" life stuff, there's always this constant vigilance that never fully goes away. A part of your mind always peeking around the corner, checking to see if the lion is back.

When someone says, "You're fine now," you want to believe them. But part of you wonders if that's really true, or if the lion is just out of sight, waiting.

Fear of recurrence isn't irrational. It's what happens when your life gets hijacked by something that doesn't play fair and doesn't come with guarantees. The best thing you can do with that fear is to name it. Share it and connect with people who've lived through their own lion fight and still hesitate while check the fridge, just in case. That's how we take some of its power away.

Not by pretending it's not there. But by saying out loud: *I remember the lion. And I'm still here.*

The Aftershocks

So you got through treatment, rang the damn bell, posed for your survivor photo, and now the world expects you to go back to "normal." But nothing about you feels normal anymore. Not your body. Not your brain. Not your nervous system that now jumps at shadows and flinches at fluorescent lights. Not the aching pause in your soul when someone casually asks, "So, are you all better now?"

The truth is, the real unraveling sometimes begins *after* the fight is over.

Dina told me, "I thought I was fine until I heard that beeping noise at the grocery store. Same tone as the IV pump. I froze in the aisle and couldn't breathe. It's been three years since treatment ended, and my body still remembers."

That's what trauma does. It stores itself in the quiet corners of your body. It sits under your skin, waits in your cells, rides shotgun even when you think you've left it behind. You can't use logic and reason your way out of it. You can't use yoga or green smoothies to beat it into submission. Because trauma doesn't speak in words, it speaks in triggers.

A smell. A sound. A phrase. A date on the calendar.

Suddenly, you're back in the chemo chair. Back in the office with the surgeon's face frozen in bad news. Back to the very moment when you realized your life would never look the same again.

And even when the scans are clear, even when you're finally declared "cancer-free," the fear still hums underneath it all.

Nadia said, "Even when the scans come back clean, I still hold my breath. It's like I'm always bracing for something bad. Cancer didn't just change my body. It completely rewired my sense of safety."

There's no expiration date on hyper-vigilance. On waking up in the night, heart pounding, because your dream tricked you back into the fight. On feeling guilty for not feeling grateful every second of the day. On standing in your own kitchen and wondering why joy feels like a stranger.

You are not crazy. You're not ungrateful. You're not broken.

You're just not done healing yet.

Some days, it's grief that blindsides you. Not just grief for the things you lost, but grief for the person you used to be. The version of you who hadn't faced all of this. Who hadn't carried this weight. Who hadn't had to grow up so fast in the face of your own mortality.

Simone said, "Everyone kept saying how lucky I was, how strong I was, but I felt so empty. Like I'd survived a fire, and now I was standing in the ashes not knowing how to rebuild."

That image, standing in the ashes, is one so many of us recognize. Because when cancer leaves, it doesn't leave things tidy. It leaves holes. Gaps. Burn marks. Silence. And you're supposed to rebuild without a blueprint, using pieces that no longer quite fit, and everyone that had helped you has gone home.

Tanya told me, "I'm not the same woman I was before cancer. I don't think I ever will be. But I'm learning to love the version of me that came out on the other side."

That's post-traumatic growth. Not the kind people wrap in a bow or call a blessing in disguise. It comes from facing the unthinkable and still finding a way to show up as the person you are now: flawed, fierce, afraid, and still standing.

The aftershocks are real. But so is your resilience.

You don't have to rush this part. You don't have to pretend you're okay. Just keep going. Even if all you do today is breathe. Even if the bravest thing you do this week is get out of bed and put on pants.

You are not alone in the fallout. And you don't have to rebuild by yourself. You just need to put one foot in front of the other.

✅ Chapter Highlights

- Fear of recurrence is a normal and common part of life after treatment. It's a trauma response rooted in real experience.

- PTSD can develop after cancer treatment, triggered by sensory reminders or upcoming scans. Naming it can be the first step toward healing.

- Long-term effects of treatment may include neuropathy, lymphedema, chemo brain, and emotional struggles. These deserve attention and care.

- Tools like journaling, grounding exercises, supportive relationships, and trauma-informed therapy can help ease fear and foster resilience.

- Ongoing diagnostic imaging, lab work, bone scans, and heart monitoring play key roles in long-term survivorship care.

🤍 Key Takeaway:

The fear of recurrence may never fully disappear, but it doesn't have to control you. Healing is not about forgetting the trauma—it's about learning to live with the scars and still choose joy, love, and peace anyway.

"Scars"

I look in the mirror at all of my scars.
I see the one on the breast of the 20 year old innocent young bride.
Told if it was malignant, the breast would come off
I said, I'd rather die.
An immature reaction to what I thought made me beautiful.
A romanticized vision of a young Juliet lying in repose.
Foolish girl, lucky girl

I look in the mirror and see the scars on my abdomen.
The ones where a scalpel sliced so delicately into the womb
And brought forth three beautiful, healthy sons.
The scars that forced a young woman to wear
the matronly one piece suit in a time of sexy string bikinis.
Vain young woman, self-conscious young woman.

I see the scar of the biopsy probe. Its dimple a small basin
catching the water that flows down from the shower spout.
I look in the mirror and see the scars
across my breast and under my arm.
The scars created when the tentacles of cancer
were carved out of my body
Carefully preserving the healthy tissue,
but distorting the remains just the same.

I look in the mirror and see the scars where children lay their little
heads,
smelling sweet and delicious,
while grandma reads a bedtime story and sings them lullabies.
I see the scars where they place their hands and tell me I feel "squishy."
The scars where they ask to see my booboos
and offer a Tinkerbell or Muppet bandaid.

I look in the mirror and see the scars of a well-loved lifetime.
Scars that brought forth life; that saved a life.
A blessed wife, and mother, and grandma.
Grateful woman, thankful woman.

~Gerry Kearney

19
Managing Recurrence & What-If Scenarios

There are few phrases more life-altering than "You have cancer." But perhaps one that cuts even deeper is: *"It's back."*

If you're reading this chapter, you may be navigating one of the most frightening moments of your life. The ground may feel unsteady. The air may feel thinner, and the hope you fought so hard to hold onto might suddenly feel out of reach again.

Please hear this: Your story may be uniquely yours, but you are not alone.

You're also not starting from scratch. You are someone who already knows how to fight. You've learned how to sit through appointments that last too long and wait for phone calls that come too late. You've figured out how to make it through chemo, scans, surgeries, and days when everything hurts, including your spirit. You've already proven how resilient and resourceful you are, even if it didn't feel like it at the time.

But this is a new chapter. And while it may be terrifying, it's also one you don't have to face the same way you did before.

This time, you know your body. You know the questions to ask. You know your worth. You've learned how to advocate for yourself, how to rest when you need to, and how to let love in when it's offered.

You're not alone in this chapter either. Now is the time to lean on every connection you have, from your medical team to your family and friends. But also, reach out to others who are walking this same path. Hold hands and face it together. There are support groups filled with people who understand your fear without needing an explanation. There are online forums, group therapy options, and communities where you can say what you're *really* feeling, without being met with pity or toxic positivity.

It's okay to scream. It's normal to grieve. And it's especially okay to say, *"I'm not ready to do this again."*

But please, keep going anyways.

And while I've been fortunate with seventeen years out from my diagnosis without recurrence, I know and understand the fear. I know what it feels like to walk into a mammogram appointment with a knot in your stomach. Every scan, every follow-up, carries a silent question: *What if it's back?* I've lived with that question for years, and I've seen others get the answer that all of us dread.

I can only imagine the devastation of hearing it a second time. I don't pretend to fully understand it, but I hold space for the weight of it. Because even without recurrence, the fear itself is real, and it's heavy.

This chapter exists to help you find your way through the chaos. We'll walk through how recurrence is confirmed, what your treatment options might look like, and how to care for your mental and emotional well-being in the process. We'll talk about second opinions, financial prep, legal planning, and palliative care, not because we've given up on hope, but because hope lives in preparedness.

You are a warrior. Tired, maybe, and definitely changed. But no less worthy of healing, support, and peace.

Let's take this one step at a time. Together.

Confirming Recurrence

When the worry creeps in, or when something doesn't feel quite right, it's natural to want answers fast. If your doctor suspects a recurrence, they'll usually order imaging like PET/CT scans, MRIs, or bone scans. Sometimes, they'll recommend a biopsy to get clear, updated pathology. It's scary, waiting for those tests and results, but it helps to know what they're looking for and why.

There are two broad categories doctors refer to: local recurrence, which means the cancer has come back in the breast, chest wall, or nearby lymph nodes, and metastatic recurrence (Stage IV), which means it has spread to other parts of your body, like the bones, lungs, or liver.

Neither diagnosis defines your worth or your strength. It's a tool to help the doctors chart the next step of your treatment path.

Stacey knows this road all too well. At 35, she faced her second breast cancer diagnosis, fourteen years after her first. "Walking into chemo the second time," she said, "I knew exactly what was coming. That made it scarier in some ways, but I also knew I could do it. I had done it before. And that gave me power."

Amber shared something similar: "I thought I was done. I did everything they told me to. But two years later, it showed up in my spine. I didn't cry right away. I just sat there thinking, 'How the hell am I supposed to do this again?'"

That's the thing about recurrence, it hits differently. There's no blissful ignorance the second time around. But there is experience. There's wisdom and power in knowing what you're capable of.

Second-Line Treatments

If it turns out the cancer has returned, your treatment plan may shift, but that doesn't mean all your options are gone. In fact, many people live meaningful, full lives after recurrence. The medical world has evolved and there are so many more tools now than there used to be.

Depending on your history and the current behavior of your cancer, your oncologist may suggest a new chemotherapy or hormone therapy, a targeted therapy that zeroes in on specific tumor traits, immunotherapy if your cancer is a good candidate, or even participation in a clinical trial.

It might feel overwhelming, but take heart, this next plan is built on everything your body has already been through and everything we now know about how cancer behaves. You're not starting over. You're building forward.

Camille put it this way: "I stopped saying 'I beat cancer.' I say 'I'm living with cancer.' Because it never really leaves you. Not when it's in your blood, and not when it's in your memory. I don't need to be a warrior every day. Some days, I'm just a woman trying to make her coffee without crying."

🐾 Palliative & Supportive Care

Let's clear something up. Palliative care is not the same as hospice. Palliative care is about quality of life. It's a medical specialty focused on easing pain, fatigue, nausea, and emotional distress, while you're still pursuing treatment. It's okay to ask for that kind of support right now.

And if the time ever comes when curative treatment isn't the goal anymore, hospice care becomes the next level of compassionate support. It's about dignity, comfort, and being surrounded by love—not wires and white coats.

Kelly was one of the women who faced metastatic recurrence.

"I kept thinking every ache was the cancer coming back," she shared. "And then one day, it was. I went from worrying to knowing. But even then, I decided to live, not only survive. I started yoga again. I changed my diet. I asked for help. And I held onto the hope that good days could still happen."

Lilli took a different path. Hers was rooted in clarity and peace: "When they told me it was back, I didn't flinch. I just asked how much time I had. I'd already done the surgeries, the chemo, the radiation. I didn't want to live whatever time I had left being poisoned again. I wanted to be with my family. To eat what I wanted. To feel the sun on my skin and laugh without being afraid."

There is no one right choice. There is only *your* choice.

🧠 Mental, Emotional & Practical Planning

There's nothing defeatist about making a plan. In fact, planning can be an incredibly empowering act. It says, *I am still here. I still have a say in how this goes.*

That might mean talking with a therapist who understands the trauma of recurrence and the layers of grief and fear that come with it. It might mean reviewing your finances—figuring out what's covered, what isn't,

226

and whether new treatments or drugs are accessible through assistance programs. It might mean updating your legal documents—like a living will or power of attorney—not because you've lost hope, but because you're making sure your wishes are known.

These steps are not a surrender. They're acts of love for yourself and your people.

When Life Logistics Shift

A new diagnosis often means your life gets rearranged, again. And that's not easy for anyone.

You might need fresh authorizations from your insurance. Updated paperwork. A shift in who takes the kids to school, who drives you to treatment, who picks up dinner.

It's okay if the ground feels wobbly. You don't need to fix everything today. Just take a look at what's changing and what help you might need. Start there. One thing at a time.

Finding Hope and Holding Onto It

Even now, you still get to choose. Maybe not what's happening inside your body, but how you move through this moment: what you eat, what feels good and nourishing, how you move, who you let into your world, and what brings you a little bit of joy or comfort each day.

Hope might look different now. That's okay. It might be smaller. Quieter. But it's still there. Sometimes it shows up in tiny victories, like getting through a scan without panic. Laughing at something ridiculous. Being able to taste your coffee again.

Give yourself permission to celebrate those wins. Let yourself feel joy, even in the middle of fear. Let your care team focus on your body, while you tend to your heart.

Second Opinions & Advanced Care Centers

If you're unsure about your next steps, or just want to explore every possible path, a second opinion can be incredibly valuable.

227

You're not being disloyal or difficult. You're being thorough. A second set of expert eyes can reveal new options, from experimental therapies to clinical trials that weren't available before.

Ask your oncologist for a summary letter or referral. Gather your records: scans, biopsy results, treatment history, into a folder or digital file. Reach out to centers that specialize in breast cancer or metastatic care. Many now offer virtual appointments if travel is tough. Getting a second is building on what you've already done, with more support in your corner.

Chapter Highlights

- Recurrence may be local (in the breast or nearby lymph nodes) or metastatic (spread to other organs). Each path comes with distinct treatment needs, but neither changes your worth or strength.

- Second-line treatments, such as new chemotherapies, targeted therapies, immunotherapy, or clinical trials, offer meaningful hope for living fully after recurrence.

- Palliative care focuses on quality of life and can begin at any stage of treatment. It is not the same as hospice, which provides compassionate care when treatment is no longer curative.

- Emotional support is vital. Therapy, support groups, and community connections help manage fear, grief, and trauma related to recurrence.

- Practical planning around finances, insurance, legal documents, and family logistics allows you to maintain a sense of control and protect your peace of mind.

- Second opinions from advanced cancer centers may uncover additional options, especially for complex or metastatic cases. Never stop advocating for yourself.

- Daily choices around movement, nutrition, joy, and community become acts of hope. Even small victories deserve to be celebrated.

💚 **Key Takeaway**

Recurrence isn't the end of your story. It's a hard, terrifying chapter, but one that you don't have to face alone or from scratch. You are wiser now. Stronger. And more than ever, you deserve hope, care, and peace.

"You may have to fight a battle more than once to win it."
—Margaret Thatcher

20
When Cancer Wins

There are no easy words for this chapter, because this is the part nobody that wants to write about. Nobody wants to talk about. And no one ever wants to live. But we owe it to the people we love to include it anyways. We have to name the fear and offer clarity in the storm. Because sometimes, cancer doesn't go away. Sometimes, it doesn't get better. And when that happens, we need just as much guidance, care, and compassion as we did in the beginning of this journey.

Resources for grief support, hospice care, and family counseling can be found in the back of this book. If you or your loved ones are struggling, please don't wait to reach out. Whether it's for yourself or a family member, these services are there to walk beside you through the loss, through the healing, and through whatever comes next.

Lilli Rabe was the kind of person who brought a little extra light into the world without even trying. She was a mother. A partner. A writer. A joyful, grounded woman who loved bright colors, soft music, and laughing at her own jokes. When her breast cancer returned, this time incurable, she sat with the truth like a friend she didn't invite but welcomed anyway.

She knew what lay ahead for her, and instead of chasing one more round of treatment that would leave her exhausted, she made a different choice. She chose time. Not just the days on the calendar, but the moments that fill them: coffee with her partner on the porch, dance parties in the kitchen with her kids, handwritten notes, and the warmth of sunlight through the window.

Hospice was not her giving up. It was her gathering in. She brought in her favorite artwork. Hung up photos of the people she loved. Played music that made her feel alive and at peace. She made her room a place to be fully seen. She asked for visitors. For honesty and friendship. For goodbyes that weren't hidden behind closed doors. She held her children's hands. She let herself cry. And she let others cry too.

She planned her memorial music and told stories she didn't want lost. She wrote notes to friends. She reminded her partner how much he was loved. She didn't pretend it wasn't happening, and she didn't want anyone else to pretend either. She faced death the way she faced life: open-hearted, creative, a little messy, and full of love.

Her story is not just about dying. It's about claiming every moment left and filling it with meaning. Lilli Rabe chose presence over fear. And it reminds us: even when cancer wins the body, it doesn't get to take the soul. Even in pain, there can be peace.

Lilli's final chapter wasn't about dying.
It was about her living in a way that honored her spirit, her family, and the love that carried her all the way through.

What Happens When Curative Treatment Ends

The moment when treatment shifts from fighting the cancer to simply caring for the person is very personal, and often filled with emotions that don't have names. Sometimes it's a hard stop, other times a slow realization. You'll feel it in conversations with your oncologist, in your body, in your spirit. When treatments stop helping or begin to cause more harm than healing, your medical team may start to talk about comfort care. That phrase alone can feel like a huge loss. But comfort care doesn't mean you've given up. This is the time for honoring what matters most: your peace, your presence, your ability to rest without suffering.

Palliative care teams step in, asking questions about your pain and your energy, your goals, your fears. They'll help manage the physical symptoms like nausea, fatigue, and shortness of breath, while also caring for the ache in your heart and the swirl of thoughts in your head. It's not a lesser kind of care. It's a gentler one. And it's every bit as important.

Questions to Ask When Time is Short

When you begin to wonder how much time is left, it's okay to ask. You're not being morbid, and you're not giving up. You're certainly not inviting death just by talking about it. You're being brave, and these are the kinds of conversations that make room for preparation and for the sacred space of saying goodbye. They allow you and your loved ones to share what matters most: the memories, laughter, forgiveness, gratitude.

Doctors may not always be able to offer a specific date or timeline, but they can usually speak in general terms. They may say weeks, months, or even longer, depending on the situation. And more importantly, they can help you understand what this next part might look like. They can give you an idea of what changes to expect in your body, in your energy, in your appetite or breathing. They can guide you through the process, step by step, so that you're not walking into the unknown alone.

Some questions you might consider asking include:
"What will this next part of the journey look like?"
"Are there any remaining treatments that might give me more good days than hard ones?"
"How should I prepare my home?"
"What support services, like hospice or palliative care, are available to help us?"
"What signs should I or my loved ones watch for?"

These conversations aren't easy. But they are acts of deep love, for yourself, for the people around you, and for the time you have left. They are gifts of clarity and courage, and they help ensure that your remaining days are shaped by intention, comfort, and dignity.

Understanding the Physical Signs of Dying

As the body begins to let go, changes tend to arrive quietly, almost imperceptibly at first. Your loved one may start sleeping more because their body is doing sacred, deep work. They may stop eating or drinking because the body no longer needs or processes fuel in the same way. You might notice their skin becoming cool to the touch, or see mottling purplish, marbled patterns, especially on the hands and feet. Breathing rhythms often change too. There may be long pauses between breaths, a soft rattle, or slower, shallower inhales.

These signs can be incredibly hard to witness. They stir up fear and helplessness, even when you understand what's happening. But most of the time, they are not signs of suffering. They are simply the body's natural way of easing out of this world. Hospice nurses are trained to

233

recognize these stages. They can walk you through what to expect, explain what's normal, and guide you gently in how to offer comfort, whether that's holding a hand, applying a cool cloth, whispering words of love, or just sitting in silence.

Being present during this time is one of the most powerful gifts you can give. Your calm presence matters. Your love matters. Even when there are no more words to say.

Offering Comfort Without Needing the Right Words

One of the most common fears people carry when someone they love is dying is this: "What if I say the wrong thing?" But in these sacred moments, it's rarely about having the perfect words. It's about showing up, exactly as you are. Sit beside them. Hold their hand, even if it's cold or still. Let your breathing slow. Light a candle. Maybe bring a familiar scent into the room like lavender, peppermint, eucalyptus, anything that once made them feel safe or soothed. You can read to them, if it feels right. A favorite poem. A passage from scripture. A worn-out novel they always returned to.

And if they don't want words, that's okay too. You don't have to fill the space with sound. Just being there is often enough. Your presence says more than any sentence could. If they speak, listen with your whole heart. If they don't, stay anyway. Sit through the quiet. Through the tears. Through the stillness. Presence is the language of love at the end of life. It says: "You're not alone. I'm here. I see you. And I'm not going anywhere."

Pain Management and the Role of Hospice

Pain does not have to be the defining experience of someone's final days. With the right care, suffering can be softened. Hospice nurses are trained in managing not just physical pain, but also breathlessness, restlessness, nausea, fear, and anxiety. They come not only with medication, but with the wisdom and skill of knowing how to read the smallest signs, how to gently reposition a weary body, how to bring peace to a troubled breath.

They monitor comfort constantly, adjusting medications as needed with compassion and skill. And they teach you, the family and caregivers, how to help by speaking gently, how to hold someone without hurting, how to recognize when it's time to just sit in stillness.

Hospice provides a way to live the final chapter with dignity and intention. It brings more than supplies like hospital beds, oxygen tanks, and comfort kits. It brings people. Aides who wash hair and change linens with grace and respect. Chaplains who pray, listen, or sit quietly in shared silence. Social workers who help you navigate the emotional, financial, and logistical weight of what's coming. Hospice is an entire team of people trained and wrapped in tenderness. A soft place to land when the road has been long.

📣 Talking About Death—Even When It's Hard

There's no easy way to begin a conversation about death. But you don't need to have all the right words. Just be honest. Speak while you still feel well enough to share your wishes. Tell your family what matters most to you. Let them know what kind of care you want and what kind of memorial would feel meaningful. Talk about who you trust to make decisions if you can't. Share your favorite songs, your hopes for your children, the stories and memories you don't want to be forgotten.

If the words won't come, try writing them down. Record a video message if that feels easier. Or ask someone you love to help put your thoughts into words. These conversations don't mean you are giving up. They're about showing and giving your love fully, even in the face of something hard. And long after you're gone, the people who love you will carry those messages with them. They will remember what you shared. They will remember that you had the courage to speak it out loud.

👶 What to Say to Children or Teens

Children and teenagers often understand more than we think. Even if no one says a word, they notice the changes. The whispered phone calls. The way grownups suddenly avoid eye contact. What they need more than anything is truth spoken gently. You might say, "My body is very sick, and the doctors can't fix it," or, "I might die soon, but I want you to know how much I love you, and that you'll never be alone."

235

Let them ask their questions. Answer as truthfully as you can. Let them cry, let them be angry, let them laugh. Kids grieve in waves. They might sob one minute and ask for ice cream the next. That doesn't mean they don't understand. It means they're doing the best they can to process something enormous. Let them help if they ask to. Offer space when they need it. Keep reminding them that no matter what happens, they are loved. They are safe. And they are not alone.

If You're Afraid to Die

It's okay to admit that you're scared. Saying, "I'm afraid," is a very normal thing. Fear in these moments is natural, and you don't have to carry it alone. Talk to someone who is able to hold that fear with you, like a nurse who's seen it before, a chaplain who knows how to listen, a therapist who understands trauma, or a friend who loves you no matter what.

Let yourself cry. Let yourself be held. You don't have to make peace with every part of this process to still find peace in the moment. Maybe it won't come from perfect closure. Maybe it will come in the stillness of someone sitting beside you, not needing to fix anything. Maybe it's in the rhythm of shared breathing. In a soft blanket. In the warmth of a hand in yours. In knowing that your life mattered. That you were deeply loved. And that your story, every messy, brave, beautiful part of it, won't be forgotten.

When the Time Comes

Not everyone gets a miracle. Not every story has a comeback. Some journeys don't end in remission or return to "normal." Some end in the slow, quiet unraveling of a life that has been lived with grit and grace, and love and pain, and everything in between.

If you're here because your cancer came back or won't go away, or because you're sitting beside someone you love who's running out of time, please hear me: there is still beauty to be found. Even here.

There's beauty in the way we soften toward each other. In the way we hold hands without needing to fix a thing. In the way we show up and are present. There is beauty in painting toenails, whispering jokes, and a meal eaten together under the sun. There's a kind of sacredness in these endings that no scan or stage number can ever quantify.

Lilli understood this in her bones. "When they told me it was back, I didn't flinch. I just asked how much time I had. I'd already done the surgeries, the chemo, the radiation. I didn't want to live whatever time I had left being poisoned again. I wanted to be with my family. To eat what I wanted. To feel the sun on my skin and laugh without being afraid."

That's a woman who knew her soul was worth listening to.

Meghan shared the story of her mother's final days. "My mom went into hospice on a Wednesday. She told me she wasn't scared, just tired. She said, 'Don't cry when I go. I'll finally get some peace.' We sat on the bed and painted our nails. Lavender. That's the last memory I have of her. She was smiling, with perfect nails, finally able to rest."

What a gift, to be loved like that at the end. To be unafraid. To be witnessed not as a patient, but as a whole, complete human being, still worthy of lavender nail polish and laughter.

And for those sitting at the bedside, aching for the right thing to say, Rachel offers this quiet truth: "Nobody teaches you how to be with someone who's dying. I kept trying to say the perfect thing, when really she just needed me to sit with her. To hold her hand and let the silence speak."

Sometimes love doesn't look like fixing. Sometimes love is simply sitting still and staying close. Sometimes it's holding a hand, adjusting a blanket, and making space for the sacred work of letting go. It can be soft. It can be music and sunlight and a room full of breath and memory. It can be a slowing down instead of a shutting off.

And when the time comes, whether it's your time, or someone else's, I hope you remember that death is not the opposite of life. It's the doorway on the far end of it. The breath that follows the last word. The gentle closing of a chapter that was always going to end.

Let it be holy. Let it be honest. Let it be whatever it needs to be.

And know this: you are not alone here either.

✔ Chapter Highlights

- Not all cancer stories end in remission. When cancer becomes terminal, care shifts from curing to comfort. Palliative and hospice care play essential roles.

- Hospice focuses on dignity and quality of life during the final stages, offering physical, emotional, and spiritual support.

- End-of-life planning includes legal documents (like living wills, advance directives, and healthcare proxies), as well as personal preparations such as letters, memorial preferences, and keepsakes.

- Caregivers also need support. Grief can begin before death, and their emotional and physical needs deserve care too.

🩶 Key Takeaway

Even when cancer takes a life, it doesn't take the love, the meaning, or the legacy left behind. Facing death with honesty, connection, and compassion can turn even the hardest goodbye into a sacred, beautiful final chapter.

"How people die remains in the memory of those who live on."
—Dame Cicely Saunders (founder of the modern hospice movement)

21
The Ones Who Hold Us Up

We often hear people say, "You're so strong," to the one going through cancer. And it's true. There is a deep, undeniable strength required to survive diagnosis, treatment, and everything in between. But there's another kind of strength that doesn't get talked about nearly enough. It doesn't wear a hospital bracelet. It doesn't have the title of "patient." It's the kind of strength that shows up to every appointment, takes notes while pretending they aren't every bit as scared, and keeps moving forward even when everything feels like it's falling apart.

This kind of strength is quiet. It makes dinner and does laundry. It drives kids to school, picks up prescriptions, and spends hours in waiting rooms trying to be the steady one. It cancels plans, rearranges work schedules, and lies awake at night wondering what comes next. It cries in the shower so no one else has to see it. It puts on a brave face in front of the kids. It holds everything together while watching the person they love fall apart. And far too often, this kind of strength goes unacknowledged. Unseen. Unthanked.

That's the caregiver.

And I want to be really honest about this part, because it's complicated. It's messy. It's full of love, but also full of heartbreak. And for many of us, it's one of the most emotionally painful pieces of the entire story.

During my treatment, I had two primary caregivers. My husband at the time, and my dear friend Tammy. They showed up in different ways. Tammy brought meals, picked up my children from school, and sat beside me when I didn't have the words to talk, but needed someone near. She gave me her weekends, her evenings, her presence. She gave me her heart. My husband, in those earlier days, managed the logistics. He made sure I ate, stayed through chemo, helped coordinate everything. He held space for me, up until he didn't.

Neither of those relationships survived my cancer journey.

And I still carry guilt. Not just for the ways they left, but for the ways I failed to see their pain. I didn't always say thank you. I didn't ask how they were coping. I didn't recognize how heavy it must have been to love me through that storm. I was so buried in my own fear, my own grief, that I didn't notice they were drowning too. I know they held resentment, because they gave so much, and still ended up feeling invisible.

Beth told me about her sister: "My sister came to every chemo appointment. She brought snacks, blankets, crossword puzzles. She made it a ritual. I don't think I could have walked through that season without her steadiness."

And Rachel shared how her best friend helped in the quietest, most healing ways: "My best friend didn't try to fix anything. She just came over and sat with me. Sometimes we didn't even talk. She'd just braid my hair or make toast. That was more healing than any card or casserole."

Arlene talked about her husband, and how caregiving took a toll even when he never said a word: "He emptied my drains without flinching. He shaved my head when the clumps started falling. He never said it out loud, but I could see the pain in his eyes. Loving someone through cancer is its own kind of grief."

I'm sharing all of this because I don't want others to fall through the same cracks. I want us to see caregivers, not just as helpers, but as people who are also struggling to find ways of navigating their own version of this trauma. Caregivers are hurting too. And if we don't acknowledge that hurt, if we leave them unsupported and unseen, it doesn't just disappear. It festers. It builds walls. It turns love into resentment.

Caregivers go through stages, just like patients do. They experience fear, grief, guilt, exhaustion, tenderness, resentment, helplessness, and love, sometimes all in a single day. But the difference is, they rarely get the permission to fall apart. They hold it in. They carry it quietly. And too often, they do it without the support they desperately need.

So this chapter is for them. For the ones behind the scenes. The ones holding the tissues, making the meals, cleaning the bathrooms, scheduling the rides, and standing by with hearts full of fear and hands always full. It's time we see them too.

📣 A Note to the Caregiver Reading This

If you're holding this book because someone you love is fighting cancer, thank you. Truly. I see you. I see the exhaustion in your eyes and the way your phone is always on low battery from constant updates and appointment reminders. I see the endless mental lists running through your head, even in the quietest moments when it looks like you're finally resting.

You might not feel like a hero. Some days you might feel frustrated or angry. Other days, the guilt might sneak in when you wish, just for a second, that things could go back to the way they were. You might not even recognize yourself anymore because your life has shifted so dramatically into someone else's survival story.

But here's what I see when I look at you: a heart that keeps showing up, over and over, even when no one is watching. A pair of hands doing the invisible, thankless labor that keeps everything going behind the scenes. A soul carrying someone else's pain in addition to your own, often without being asked and without complaint.

You are not just a helper. You are not a background character in this story. You are part of it. And you deserve to be seen.

I know you're tired. Not just physically, but deep in your spirit. I know that when people check in, they ask about the patient. They seldom how you are. So let me say what maybe no one else has said yet: you matter. Your exhaustion matters. Your pain, your fear, your grief, it all matters.

You're allowed to feel overwhelmed, and to say, "I'm not okay either." You have needs and limits, even when someone else's crisis seems bigger. If anyone tries to make you feel like you have to justify your emotions, please remember this: cancer doesn't follow the rules. Neither do the emotions it drags along with it.

Let this chapter be a breath. A soft place to land for just a moment. You are constantly giving care, but you deserve a rest as well. You deserve to be supported, held, and reminded that you are not invisible. You are loved. You are needed. And you are not alone.

⌚ When You've Been on Both Sides

There's something I don't hear talked about enough, and I want to say it here because it's important: sometimes, being the one going through cancer can feel easier than being the one watching someone go through it. That may sound strange, even backwards, but having lived on both sides, I believe it's true.

When you're the patient, your role is clear. You're the one receiving treatment, the one sitting in the chemo chair, the one being poked, scanned, and monitored. It's terrifying, but it's defined. People expect you to fall apart. They prepare for it. You're given space to rest, to receive help, and to not be okay.

But when you're the caregiver, there's no clear path. Just a set of unspoken expectations. Keep it together. Stay strong. Anticipate every need. Hold space for someone else's fear, even when your own is eating you alive. And the worst part is that you don't have any control. You're watching someone you love suffer, and there's nothing you can do to stop it. That helplessness, standing by while the person you care about is in pain, messes with your head and your heart. It wears down your body and quietly chips away at your spirit.

It's hard to talk about and you'll probably keep to yourself how heavy it feels and how much it's wearing you down. You won't want to take up space or shift the focus. But staying silent doesn't make the pain disappear. It just buries it deeper. But, buried pain doesn't stay buried. It shows up later in burnout, in resentment, in numbness, or in the moments when everything finally falls apart.

So I want you to know: it *is* about you too. You are allowed to have emotions, even messy ones. You are allowed to say, "This is hard for me too." Because it is. And saying it out loud might just be the first step toward the care and healing you deserve.

There's nothing selfish about needing support. Everyone needs some kind of help once in a while in their lives. There's nothing wrong with asking for it, and accepting it!

242

Let's start there.

🧠 The Emotional Toll of Caring

Caregiving is one of the most generous and emotionally demanding roles a person can take on. Most of the time, it happens behind the scenes, quietly and without applause. There are no medals handed out for waking up at 3 a.m. to hold someone's hand through a panic attack. No award ceremonies for making sure the insurance forms are filled out correctly while swallowing your own tears. And yet, you keep showing up. Over and over. Because love tells you to. Because purpose drives you. Because adrenaline gets you through the first part.

But as days turn into weeks and weeks stretch into months, the toll becomes undeniable. You might start to feel anger bubble up. Anger that your life has been put on hold, that your needs have taken a backseat. And almost immediately, that anger is followed by guilt. How can you be angry when they're the one with cancer? You might find yourself grieving, not just for the version of your loved one who used to laugh more, but for the version of yourself who once had space to think about dreams, passions, plans of your own.

These emotions aren't wrong. They're not selfish. They're not something to be ashamed of. They're perfectly natural feelings. And yet, so many caregivers try to push those feelings down. You tell yourself, "They don't get a break from cancer, so I shouldn't either." You convince yourself that rest is a luxury. That laughter or joy should be postponed until everything is okay again. But that's a lie cancer whispers to you. And it will leave you hollow if you keep believing it.

Your pain doesn't take away from theirs. Your exhaustion doesn't mean you're weak. It means you're living inside a storm. And taking a breath for yourself, stepping outside for fresh air, sleeping in, watching a show that makes you laugh, doesn't mean you're abandoning them. It means you love them enough to want to show up whole and ready to help.

💬 For Patients: Don't Forget Your People

When you're deep in treatment, everything narrows. Your world shrinks down to pain management, medication schedules, and simply making it through each day. You're overwhelmed. I remember being in that place,

243

exhausted, scared, emotionally shredded, and how easy it was to disappear into my own survival. I often called it my bubble. But here's something I've learned: the people beside you are just surviving, too.

I didn't always see that. I didn't think to ask how my caregivers were holding up. I didn't check in on their feelings and fears. I didn't say thank you nearly as often as I should have. And even now, years later, I carry a quiet regret for that.

So if you're the one being cared for, I hope you'll hear this gently: your caregiver is carrying a heavy load, too. Please check in on them. Give them permission for care for themselves. Ask how they're feeling. Let them vent. Let them cry if they need to. If you have more than one support person, don't let it all fall on one set of shoulders. Let someone else bring dinner. Let your best friend sit with you while your spouse gets out of the house for an afternoon. Let your teenager help with the laundry, even if the towels end up folded the "wrong" way. Small breaks matter.

When your energy is low, you might not have much to give. But a simple thank you, spoken with intention, written in a note, whispered with a hand squeeze, can change so much. That acknowledgment can be the balm that keeps your caregiver going.

Because caregivers aren't just helping you get through treatment. They're going through the emotions, too. And the more seen and appreciated they feel, the lighter the load becomes for both of you.

How to Support the Ones Who Support You

Your spouse. Your sister. Your best friend. Your grown child. Whoever has stepped into the role of caregiver, they're in it with you. One of the most meaningful gifts you can give them is permission. Permission to rest. Permission to step back without guilt. Permission to not be perfect. So many caregivers push themselves beyond exhaustion because they think they have to. Remind them, gently and often, that they don't have to hold everything on their own. They're already doing more than enough.

If possible, try to share the load. Even small shifts can make a difference. Use a shared calendar to coordinate appointments. Set up a meal train with friends or neighbors. Create a small care team of three or four people who can rotate tasks like picking up groceries or checking in. Don't let it all land on one person's shoulders. Even superheroes need to wash their capes once in a while.

When you see your caregiver starting to fray at the edges looking tired, short-tempered, or like they're carrying too much, don't just say "thank you." Show it. Let them go be something other than a caregiver for a while. Take off the superhero cape and care for themselves while you call a friend to step in. It's okay.

They may not say it, but they need that kind of grace. And if they begin to lose themselves in your story, forgetting that their needs matter too, remind them that this is their story, too. Their pain, their love, their exhaustion, and their healing all deserve space. Their presence is not just a background detail. It's part of the heartbeat that keeps this whole journey working like a well-oiled machine.

✔️ Chapter Highlights

- Caregivers carry emotional, physical, and mental burdens that often go unseen and unspoken.

- Their experience is just as real and deserves attention, compassion, and support.

- Unchecked stress can turn into resentment, which can damage relationships over time.

- Patients can help by checking in, sharing responsibilities, expressing gratitude, and letting others help.

💟 Key Takeaway

Behind every person facing cancer is someone holding them up. Their role is sacred. Their pain is real. And their healing matters too. Caregivers are not background characters in this story, they are part of the heartbeat. And they deserve to be cared for, seen, and supported just as much.

"Make your mess your message."
— *Robin Roberts; publicly documented treatment, focusing on faith and strength*

22

Seen & Strong:
Navigating Breast Cancer as a Man

When Gerald first felt the lump beneath his skin, he ignored it. He figured it was just a cyst, maybe a knot in the muscle. Breast cancer didn't even cross his mind. "That's not something men get," he thought.

So he waited. Six months passed in silence. By the time he finally saw a doctor, the lump had grown large enough to raise concern. Even then, the nurse filling out his intake form seemed unsure. "You mean chest mass, right?" she asked.

And that's how it started, the questioning, the invisibility, the subtle ways the system reminded him he didn't quite belong. Even the hospital gown felt wrong: floral print, soft pinks, clearly designed for someone else's body. The waiting room was filled with women. The brochures, the posters, the language, none of it included him. It felt like having a disease no one believed he could get.

Then came the biopsy. Then the diagnosis: Invasive Ductal Carcinoma. Breast cancer.

Gerald was stunned. Suddenly, he was a man with a diagnosis that didn't seem to belong to him. People had no idea what to say. Some friends offered comments like, "Well, at least it's not prostate cancer." A few laughed awkwardly. Others avoided the topic altogether. The pink ribbon that symbolized awareness and hope didn't feel like it was meant for him. He didn't see himself reflected in any support groups. Even the word "survivor" felt like it belonged to someone else.

Joe K. felt that same disconnect: "I was diagnosed at 67. I'd never even *heard* of men getting breast cancer. I didn't want to tell anyone at first. I felt embarrassed. Like my diagnosis was some kind of mistake. It took me a while to say it out loud to other people. But once I did, I found out I wasn't alone after all."

Richard shared the moment that drove his isolation home: "I walked into that waiting room and it was all pink. There were only women in there. I kept thinking, 'Do I even belong here?' But the tumor in my chest didn't care that I was a man. It just grew anyway."

In the same way that cancer doesn't care what you have planned on your calendar, cancer also doesn't care about gender. And neither should your support.

It took time, but eventually Gerald found others, mostly online, who had walked the same road. Other men who had heard the same diagnosis. Who had felt the same isolation. They weren't large in number, but they were strong in spirit. In their stories, he found understanding and strength. And now, he shares his own story with others online, because men do get breast cancer. And they deserve to be seen as well.

◎˙ What Men Should Know

Breast cancer is often thought of as a women's disease, but men have breast tissue too. And yes, that tissue can develop cancer. In the United States, about 1 in every 100 people diagnosed with breast cancer is male. It's unusual, but it happens. And for many men, diagnosis comes later than it should. Not because they weren't paying attention, but because no one ever told them to.

There's no standard screening protocol for men like there is for women. No yearly mammograms unless you're considered to be high-risk. But that doesn't mean you should ignore changes in your chest. If you notice a lump, swelling, nipple discharge, discomfort, or changes in the shape of your chest, don't brush it off. You know your body. Trust what it's telling you. Speak up. You deserve to be taken seriously.

If you have a family history of breast, ovarian, pancreatic, or prostate cancer, talk to your doctor about genetic counseling. Inherited mutations like BRCA2 can significantly raise the risk of breast cancer in men. Knowing your status can shape your care plan, and help protect your children and siblings, too.

Emotionally, this journey can feel incredibly lonely. Most support groups, educational materials, and media stories don't reflect men's experiences. That doesn't make your diagnosis less valid. It doesn't make you less masculine. And it absolutely doesn't mean you have to walk this alone. Finding the right kind of support, like a therapist who understands men's health, a partner who listens without judgment, or an online brotherhood of survivors, can make a world of difference.

Because healing doesn't come from strength alone.
It comes from being seen. And you deserve to be seen.

Understanding Risk

Breast cancer in men is rare, but that doesn't mean it's impossible. And when it does happen, it often takes people by surprise, not just the men diagnosed, but their doctors, families, and friends as well. Most men who are diagnosed are over the age of 60, but it can happen earlier, especially when certain risk factors are present.

A family history of breast or ovarian cancer is one of the strongest indicators, particularly when tied to inherited mutations like BRCA2. These genetic changes can significantly increase the risk of developing breast cancer, and knowing your family's health history can be an important tool in early detection. If multiple members of your family have faced breast, ovarian, or even prostate cancer, it's worth talking to your doctor about genetic counseling.

There are other contributing factors as well. Past radiation exposure to the chest, perhaps from a previous cancer treatment, can increase the likelihood of developing breast cancer later in life. Liver disease, which alters hormone metabolism, or other conditions that disrupt the balance of estrogen and testosterone, may also play a role. Carrying excess body weight can shift hormone levels in ways that raise risk, particularly through higher levels of estrogen. And in rare cases, men with Klinefelter syndrome, which is a genetic condition in which a man is born with an extra X chromosome, may face a significantly higher risk due to increased estrogen levels and reduced testosterone.

But here's what's important to remember: having risk factors doesn't mean you're destined to get cancer. And not having risk factors doesn't mean you can't. It just means paying attention to your body matters. Noticing a change and being willing to speak up, even when it feels awkward or uncertain, can make all the difference. Early detection saves lives. And being proactive about your health is one of the most important things you can do.

💬 What Male Survivors Say

"They told me I had breast cancer, and my first reaction was, 'Are you sure?' I didn't even know that was a thing for men." — David, 62

"It's pink everything. But I'm not here for the color, I'm here to live." — Paul, 57

"Once I found other guys like me, I didn't feel so ashamed. I realized I wasn't weak. I was just one of the unlucky few. And I could still fight." — Kevin, 49

These voices remind us that while male breast cancer is often invisible in the public eye, it's very real, and survivable. What they need is inclusion. Recognition. And a space to be vulnerable and supported.

👥 Finding the Right Support

Being a man with breast cancer can feel like being invisible in a room full of people. The diagnosis alone is hard enough. But then comes the pink everything, the brochures covered in photos of women, the support groups that don't speak your language. It starts to feel like the entire system was built without you in mind.

I am acutely aware of how lonely breast cancer can feel for a woman. I can't even imagine the loneliness involved when a man has breast cancer. Surrounding yourself with people that understand what you are going through has to be difficult. It's important to find a community that sees and understands your experiences.

The Male Breast Cancer Coalition is one of the strongest communities out there. Their website, malebreastcancercoalition.org, shares powerful survivor stories, creates safe places for connection, and advocates for greater awareness and inclusion in both medical and public spaces. Another resource, zerobreastcancer.org, offers gender-inclusive information that can help men better understand what to expect during treatment and recovery.

Many men find comfort in smaller, more private places as well, like online support groups, forums, or Facebook communities where they can ask honest questions, speak freely, and vent their frustrations without worrying about judgment. These spaces might not be loud, but they are safe. And they are filled with people who get it.

If you're a caregiver to a man with breast cancer, your presence matters. But so does the way you show up. Try not to focus only on the medical facts or jump straight into problem-solving. Meet him emotionally. Hold space for the fear, the grief, and the frustration. Don't expect stoicism. Don't assume strength has to look a certain way. Let him feel what he's feeling, and allow him to be real and express those feelings in a safe environment, without needing to be fixed. Being human comes first. Healing starts there.

Questions Worth Asking

When preparing for appointments, it can help to consider some of the unique aspects of being a man with breast cancer. Ask your doctor how imaging procedures like mammograms or ultrasounds are handled for men, and what you can expect during those appointments. These things are often designed for female anatomy, so knowing how they'll be adapted for you can help ease discomfort or anxiety.

You may also want to ask about genetic testing, especially if you have a family history of cancer. Mutations like BRCA2 can increase the risk for breast cancer in men and can also carry implications for your children's health. A positive result doesn't just shape your treatment, it informs your entire family how to move forward.

Ask about the side effects of chemo, radiation, and especially hormone therapy. For men, these treatments can have vastly different physical and emotional effects. It's okay to talk about what that might mean for your energy levels, your libido, your mental health, or even your sense of identity.

Most importantly, ask about connection. Are there support groups or mentorship programs specifically for men that your care team can recommend? What about referring you to others who have been where you are? Because no matter how strong you are, you don't have to navigate this alone.

Recovery isn't only about healing your body. It's rebuilding your sense of self as well. Your voice matters. Your experience matters. And there is room for you here.

Did You Know?

Sometimes, hearing about a famous face who's been through the same thing can make the road ahead feel a little less lonely. These well-known men didn't just face breast cancer, they spoke up about it. Richard Roundtree, Peter Criss, and Matthew Knowles all used their platforms to raise awareness, encourage early detection, and break the silence around male breast cancer. Their words carry weight, reminding other men that speaking out can save lives. Whether it's Roundtree's "Breast cancer is not gender specific," Criss's "Don't be afraid, and don't sit around playing macho," or Knowles's warning that "Hiding it can be deadly," their messages are clear: you're not alone, and your voice matters.

- **Richard Roundtree** – Actor (*Shaft*), diagnosed in 1993.

- **Peter Criss** – Founding drummer of KISS, diagnosed in 2008.

- **Rod Roddy** – *The Price is Right* announcer, diagnosed in 2001.

- **Edward Brooke** – Former U.S. Senator, diagnosed in 2002.

- **Monty Python's Terry Gilliam** – Diagnosed in 2009.

- **Matthew Knowles** – Music executive (Beyoncé's father), diagnosed in 2019.

- **James Michael Tyler** – Actor (*Friends*' Gunther), diagnosed in 2018 (had prostate cancer as well, but publicly supported male breast cancer awareness).

Chapter Highlights

- Men can and do get breast cancer. While it's rare, it affects thousands every year in the U.S.

- Because of stigma and lack of public awareness, men are often diagnosed later, leading to more advanced disease.

- Risk factors include age, family history (especially BRCA2), hormone imbalances, radiation exposure, and certain genetic conditions.

- Emotional support and connection are essential. Finding male-specific or inclusive spaces can make a life-changing difference.

- Caregivers can offer deeper support by acknowledging the emotional toll, using gender-neutral resources, and validating the full range of feelings.

💜 **Key Takeaway**

Men with breast cancer are not rare stories. They are real people, often unheard, but never alone. Your diagnosis does not define your masculinity. With awareness, early detection, and the right kind of support, healing is not only possible, it's powerful.

"Don't be afraid, and don't sit around playing macho."
— Peter Criss; encouraged men to speak about breast lumps and get early treatment

23
Genetics, Family, & the Power of Information

My aunt was diagnosed with breast cancer when she was just 29 years old. This was back in the 1980s, when treatment was far more brutal, knowledge was limited, and the idea of survivorship looked very different than it does today. But she made it. She survived. And now, in her 60s, she's still here. She became my hero during my own diagnosis, living proof that survival was possible.

When I started treatment, my doctors asked about family history. Because no one in my immediate family had been diagnosed, my aunt's experience was considered "distant" and less relevant. Still, they ordered genetic testing.

The first time I was tested, it was through a university program I qualified for. The results came back negative. No BRCA mutation. No red flags. No obvious reason to worry. About 15 later, I decided to test again, this time through my OB-GYN. Once again, the results came back negative.

But even with two negative tests, I remain watchful. Not just for myself, but for my daughter.

She's 24 now. My only biological child. And even though I haven't tested positive for any of the known genes, science is still unfolding. There are genetic markers researchers may not have discovered yet. And I want her to be ready. Not fearful, but informed. That's why I talk with her openly. I encourage her to stay educated. I remind her that a negative result today doesn't guarantee anything forever.

She's already started getting annual mammograms. We don't live in fear. We live in readiness. I've given her all the information I can, and that knowledge gives us both power.

What Is Genetic Testing for Breast Cancer?

Genetic testing is a tool that helps identify inherited mutations. They are tiny changes in your DNA that can increase your risk for certain types of cancer, especially breast and ovarian cancer. The most well-known of these are BRCA1 and BRCA2, but many modern tests now screen for dozens of additional genes that may also influence your risk. Genes like PALB2, CHEK2, ATM, and others are becoming more understood, and new discoveries continue to reshape what we know about hereditary cancer.

Testing is typically done using either blood or saliva, and there are a variety of ways to access it. Some people go through a genetic counselor or specialist. Others are tested by their OB-GYN or through high-risk breast clinics. University research programs sometimes offer free or low-cost testing if you qualify. And now, at-home kits have made testing more accessible, although it's always a good idea to follow up with a healthcare provider to interpret the results accurately.

But keep in mind, it's not just about getting tested. It's about what you do with the results that really can make a difference. A positive genetic test result doesn't mean you *will* get cancer. But it does mean that your risk is elevated, and that knowledge can shape your care plan. Remember that you have choices, and it's your job to advocate for your own health care. You might choose to start earlier screenings, learn more about preventive surgeries, or ask your doctor about medication that can help reduce your risk. A negative result doesn't mean you're in the clear forever either. It simply means that no currently known mutations were found. Science is still evolving, and there's still so much we don't fully understand.

That's why context matters. Your family history, your personal health, your gut instincts, they all play a role. Genetic testing is a piece of the puzzle, but not the whole picture. It can provide clarity, and sometimes, it can bring peace of mind. But it should always come with conversations with your doctor, educating yourself on your choices, and learning about your risks before making decisions about what comes next. When it comes to cancer, preparation is one of the few things we *can* control.

Why Repeat Testing Matters

Genetic science doesn't stand still. What we knew five years ago has already been expanded, refined, and rewritten. New mutations are discovered. Panels become broader. Testing methods improve. That's why repeating your genetic testing every few years, especially if you previously tested negative, can offer fresh insight.

You're staying current, and that means staying empowered, because the more we know, the more options we have. Options for prevention, for early detection, and for guiding our daughters and our sons. And that gives more than just peace of mind. It can be lifesaving.

Questions Around Genetic Testing

Before moving forward with testing, it helps to ask the right questions. What kind of panel will be used: a basic test or a more comprehensive one? What should the next step be if the results are positive? Or if they're negative, but you still have a strong family history? Should your children or siblings be tested too?

Maggie put it simply: "The hardest part wasn't the blood draw, it was the waiting. I kept thinking, 'If it's positive, what does that mean for my daughters? For my sister?' I wasn't scared for me. I was scared for all of them."

Some tests are covered by insurance. Others may have financial aid options. Be sure to talk to your insurance company about what they cover, so you know what you're getting in to.

As more genetic markers are discovered, you may also wonder how often to test again. A genetic counselor or high-risk clinic can help you navigate these decisions with compassion and clarity.

Caring for the Next Generation: Prevention & Surveillance

Genetic testing can create a ripple effect throughout your family. When a mutation is found, it's common to recommend what's called cascade testing, which offers close relatives the chance to be tested too.

Julie shared what that moment felt like: "I didn't get tested until after my double mastectomy. When the BRCA results came back positive, I

257

remember feeling this strange combination of grief and relief. At least now I had answers. But it also meant my nieces needed to be tested. That wrecked me."

This shouldn't be about scaring people. It should be viewed as offering them knowledge. If a child or sibling carries the same mutation, their medical team can begin early, personalized surveillance. That might include regular mammograms, MRIs, or ultrasounds, often starting years before a typical screening schedule would recommend. These early check-ins are meant to watch each loved one carefully, so that if something ever pops up, it can be caught early, when treatment will have the most impact.

In some cases, people with higher genetic risk may choose preventive medications or even surgeries to reduce their chances of developing cancer. These decisions are incredibly personal. There's no one-size-fits-all path. What matters is being informed, supported, and given the freedom to choose what feels right for your body and your future.

Lara's choice was one made with clarity and love: "I chose to get tested before surgery. My mom died at 47. I didn't want to guess. When the results came back positive for BRCA1, I knew I was doing the right thing. It made the decision to remove both breasts a little easier. It was still hard, but my mind was clearer."

Talking to someone at a high-risk breast clinic or a gynecologic oncology team can offer the specialized guidance needed to navigate these choices. Discuss who would best help you in your situation with your primary care doctor. You don't have to figure this out alone.

Helping the Next Generation: Talking to Children

One of the hardest parts of managing genetic risk is figuring out how to talk about it with your kids. But here's what I've learned: you don't have to share every detail all at once. You can give information in small, honest, age-appropriate ways that empower rather than frighten.

You might say something like, "This doesn't mean you'll get cancer. It just means we're going to stay ahead of it together." Or, "Getting screened early isn't something to fear, it's something to be proud of. It means we're informed and taking care of ourselves."

Framing these conversations around strength, awareness, and choice can help the next generation see testing as a tool, not a threat hanging over their heads.

💬 Voices from the Journey

"I tested negative for BRCA, but something told me to stay on top of screening. I'm glad I did. My cancer was caught early." — Lauren, 40

"Genetics aren't destiny. They're just one part of the puzzle. Early detection saved my life." — Marina, 46

✅ Chapter Highlights

- Genetic testing can help identify inherited mutations that increase breast cancer risk, including BRCA1 and BRCA2.

- A negative test doesn't mean zero risk. It means that science hasn't found every answer yet, and it's still evolving.

- Repeating testing every few years can reveal new information and open doors to more proactive care.

- Cascade testing gives close family members the chance to understand their own risk and make informed decisions.

- Early surveillance—including MRIs, mammograms, and specialist care—can detect issues sooner and save lives.

- Conversations with children about risk can be empowering when approached with honesty, reassurance, and love.

💜 Key Takeaway

Genetic testing is creating a legacy of knowledge, strength, and choice for those who come after you. You're passing down wisdom and teaching your loved ones to advocate for themselves.

"1 in 8 women get breast cancer. Today, I'm the one."
—Julia Louis-Dreyfus; used humor and social media to share her journey; supported healthcare access

24
In Harmony: A Holistic Approach to Healing

Elena's healing journey didn't begin with her breast cancer diagnosis. It began decades earlier. Twenty years before, she had survived a violent attack that left her with spinal injuries and traumatic brain damage. From that point on, even the mildest medications triggered severe and debilitating side effects. So when doctors recommended a double mastectomy followed by years of hormone-blocking therapy, Elena knew in her heart, and in her body, that she wouldn't be able to withstand it.

But instead of rejecting doctors or turning her back on science, Elena chose a different path. She became a student of her own healing. She cleared processed foods from her kitchen. She swapped out chemical-based products for gentler, plant-based ones. She walked barefoot in the grass, spent time sitting in the sunshine, and built a rhythm of intentional stillness. Over the next few years, she created a lifestyle rooted in gentleness, drawing on herbs, clean nutrition, movement, and spiritual connection.

She never saw this as a rejection of treatment. She saw it as her body's best chance to stay in balance.

Today, she credits this holistic way of living with helping her body stay steady and keeping her cancer in check. Her story isn't a prescription. It's an invitation to stay curious. I'm not a doctor, and I'm not here to give medical advice. What I can offer is a way to ask questions. A reminder that you have options. A nudge to work with your care team to find what makes sense for *your* body.

Elena's story is one reminder among many that healing isn't one-size-fits-all. There's more than one way to research hope.

A Gentle Reminder

Nothing in this chapter is meant to replace your medical care. Think of these ideas as invitations to explore. Always weigh the pros and cons. Look into peer-reviewed research. And partner with clinicians who are open to integrative conversations.

If your current doctor isn't listening, it's okay to find one who will. You deserve a healthcare team that treats you like a whole person, not just a diagnosis.

What is Alternative or Complementary Medicine?

These terms are often used interchangeably, but they mean very different things.

- **Complementary** therapies are used *with* conventional treatment.

- **Alternative** therapies are used *instead of* conventional treatment.

This chapter is focused on safe, supportive approaches that work *alongside* medical care, and are not recommended as replacements.

Reframing Illness as a Call to Rebalance

When you hear the word "illness," it's easy to think of something broken. Something that needs to be fixed or fought. But some healers, like Dr. Richard Schulze, offer a different way of looking at it.

What if illness is your body's way of waving a flag, signaling that something's out of alignment?

One of the best mantras I've heard is simple: Stop doing what makes you sick. Start doing what makes you healthy.

You don't have to flip your entire life upside down, but pause long enough to ask, What's one small thing I can do differently today? Maybe it's swapping a packaged snack for a handful of blueberries. Stepping outside barefoot for five quiet minutes. Sipping calming tea while you breathe a little deeper. Tiny, intentional shifts might not look like much, but over time, they can help change everything.

If you're looking for a place to start, you might explore books like *There Are No Incurable Diseases* by Dr. Schulze or *Chris Beat Cancer* by Chris Wark. You don't have to agree with everything in them, but let them spark some curiosity in you. Provide you a place to start.

🍎 Nourishing the Body with Simplicity

Eating well doesn't have to mean suddenly going vegan or turning your kitchen into a science lab. Many of the world's healthiest communities, like those in the Blue Zones, or at Uchee Pines in Alabama, keep things incredibly simple.

Beans, greens, seasonal vegetables, fruits, rice, and whole grains make up the core of their meals. These aren't restrictive diets, but rather abundant ones, built around what gives the body energy instead of what takes it away.

One philosophy you may come across is *mucusless eating*, a concept introduced by Arnold Ehret. The idea is that processed and heavy foods leave behind a sticky residue in the body, while fruits and leafy greens help clean it out.

Some people try one day a week of just fruit while others swap a heavy meal for a green juice now and then. It doesn't have to be all or nothing. You're not on a fast or a cleanse. You're learning what helps your body.

✏️ What Detox Can Look Like in Real Life

"Detox" often brings to mind punishing juice fasts or pricey kits that promise overnight miracles. But in Dr. Schulze's work, it looks completely different. He talks about gentle, intentional stages that support digestion, liver and kidney function, and help your body clear out what it no longer needs. It's a process rooted in care, not restriction.

Many people describe clearer skin, steadier moods, or improved digestion, even after trying just one piece of a detox protocol. Maybe it's a morning herbal drink. Maybe it's a soothing digestive tea before bed. The goal isn't to force your body into anything. It's to work *with* it, not against it.

And detox doesn't just happen in the kitchen.

During chemo, I was told not to use traditional antiperspirant. Instead, they handed me a salt crystal. It was a smooth, solid rock I'd wet and rub under my arms. It didn't stop the sweat or the smell, but I understood the idea. They wanted my body to keep releasing what it needed to let go of.

While research hasn't definitively proven a link between aluminum-based deodorants and breast cancer, many people still choose to switch to more natural personal care products. And that's a valid choice. When your system already feels overloaded, you may want fewer chemicals interacting with it. You want less fragrance, and gentler ingredients in your daily routine.

If you're thinking about making changes, you don't have to toss everything out all at once. Start small. You might find your skin responds better to body lotions without artificial fragrance. Look for calming ingredients like calendula, oat, or aloe. If your scalp is sensitive during hair regrowth, try a sulfate-free shampoo. Even toothpaste can feel intense during chemo, so some people switch to herbal blends that are milder on the mouth. And if you're spending time outside, mineral-based sunscreens made with zinc or titanium may be more soothing for healing skin.

Start small. Try only one product at a time to see how your body reacts. You don't have to earn a gold star for using all-natural everything. Simply tune in and support your body in the way that feels most compassionate and manageable for you. Sometimes, it's as simple as drinking more water and taking a deep breath.

🍵 Sipping Your Way to Strength: Herbs & Teas

Herbal teas aren't just cozy, they can be helpful and supportive to your delicate system. In Traditional Chinese Medicine, herbs like astragalus and reishi are used to build resilience and strengthen the immune system. Green tea is packed with antioxidants and may offer a gentle energy lift. Jiaogulan and reishi are considered adaptogens, meaning they help the body respond to stress with more stability and grace.

Even something as simple as a nightly cup of chamomile or tulsi can offer grounding and comfort, like a hug from the inside out. Remember to discuss any new herbs with your doctor first, however, so they don't interact with any medications you're currently taking. Some can even render your medications useless, so be sure to ask!

Kathy didn't expect much when she started incorporating changes into her daily routine: "My daughter was into energy work and convinced me to try Reiki. I didn't think it would do anything, but after each session, I slept better. I also drank this awful-tasting tea every day that she swore by. Who knows if it helped physically, but emotionally it gave me something to control. And that helped."

☀ Supporting Healing Beyond the Physical

True healing goes beyond scans and lab results. It's also emotional and spiritual. It lives in the way we speak to ourselves, what we believe about our self worth, and how deeply connected we feel to others.

Denise found surprising relief in an ancient practice: "Acupuncture helped with my neuropathy more than anything else. I still saw my oncologist, and still did chemo, but adding that layer helped me feel like I wasn't just enduring cancer, I was actively healing."

Another beautiful tool is thermal baths. Soaking in warm water, around 102 to 104°F, for about 20 minutes, followed by quiet rest, can do wonders for your nervous system. It's been shown to support immunity, ease joint pain, and improve sleep. And let's be honest, sometimes there's nothing more healing than sliding into warm water and just letting your body exhale.

Maria created a ritual that fed her soul: "Every night, I lit a candle, said the same prayer, and wrote down one thing I still loved about my body. It became a sacred ritual. Western medicine saved me, but these little moments helped my sanity."

Other gentle, body-based supports include:
Stepping into the morning sun, even for just ten minutes, to lift your

mood and support vitamin D levels.

Walking barefoot on the grass, sand, or soil, a practice called grounding, which can reduce inflammation and help your body sleep more soundly.

Spiritual grounding, whether through prayer, meditation, affirmations, or moments of stillness, can offer a kind of nourishment that goes beyond the physical.

🌍 Longevity Lessons from the Blue Zones

Netflix has a documentary called *Live to 100: Secrets of the Blue Zones*, and it's absolutely worth watching. It explores areas of the world where people regularly live long, healthy lives, well past one hundred, and digs into what they eat, how they move, and the deep sense of purpose and community that seem to hold it all together. It's interesting to learn about their quality of life, and the lessons we can take from it when we think about healing, balance, and the choices that help us feel truly alive.

Some well known Blue Zone areas of the world include Okinawa, Sardinia, Nicoya, and Ikaria. These people aren't just surviving to 100, they're living *well*.

They eat simply, building meals around vegetables, beans, herbs, and healthy fats. They move naturally, not in gyms, but through gardening, walking, and daily chores. Their days are filled with social connection, purpose, and moments of rest. They laugh. They pray. They belong to a community.

You don't need to move across the globe to learn from them. The takeaway is this: health is rooted in the small, meaningful things. Nourish your body with simple food, connect with people who lift you up, and move with joy and purpose. Find a reason to get up in the morning. It's so important to find balance and joy in your life.

! A Word of Caution

Just because something is "natural" doesn't always mean it's safe. Some herbs, supplements, or practices can interfere with chemo, radiation, or hormone therapy.

Before you begin anything new, ask:

- Does this therapy interfere with my treatment?

- Is it supported by evidence or reliable stories?

- Who's guiding or administering it, and how are they qualified?

- How will I know if it's helping?

Always talk to your care team, and steer clear of any practice that tells you to abandon medical care completely.

Voices from the Journey

"Acupuncture helped me keep my appetite when nothing else worked." — Nina, 51
"Reiki didn't heal my cancer, but it helped me connect to my body again. That mattered to me." — Tasha, 37
"Meditation gave me back a sense of control. It didn't cure me, but it calmed me." — Elena

Chapter Highlights

- Complementary therapies like nutrition, herbs, movement, and spiritual practices can support healing **alongside** conventional treatment.

- Holistic healing is about nourishing the whole self: body, mind, and spirit.

- Everyday practices like grounding, journaling, sipping herbal tea, or switching to gentler personal care products can create meaningful shifts in how you feel.

- Resources like *Chris Beat Cancer*, and *There Are No Incurable Diseases*, can provide education, encouragement, and connection.

- Your healing path is your own. Curiosity, kindness toward your body, and trust in your instincts matter more than doing everything "right."

🤍 Key Takeaway

Your healing journey should be about building a life that feels nourishing and true to you. Whether you're adding more vegetables to your plate, swapping out a product, sipping tea before bed, or sitting quietly in the sun, every small choice to care for yourself matters. You don't have to choose between science and soul. You can honor both. The path to healing is yours to shape, and it begins by listening to the quiet wisdom of your own body.

"A long healthy life is no accident. It begins with good genes, but it also depends on good habits."
— *Dan Buettner*

25
When Healing Meets Red Tape

I was lucky in this area, and I'll be the first to say that. Because my husband was active duty military, I was covered by TRICARE during my diagnosis and treatment. And after my divorce, when I transitioned into post-treatment care, I used the VA. I never had to fight for coverage, argue over billing, or chase down pre-authorizations like so many others do.
But through friends, fellow survivors, and stories shared in waiting rooms, I've seen just how stressful the administrative side of cancer can be. The insurance. The copays. The referrals and denied claims. It can feel like a second full-time job. And it's exhausting.

So while I didn't personally walk that path, I want to hold space for those who have. I want to help you navigate it, because your energy should go toward healing, not arguing with insurance reps. You deserve care without confusion. Help without hassle. And peace without paperwork piled on top of your pain.

The Insurance Maze

One of the most common hurdles people face during cancer treatment isn't just the illness, it's the insurance. Bills arrive in waves. Some make sense. Others seem completely disconnected from the care you received. You might get three different statements for the same appointment. You might find yourself wondering if you missed something, or if they did.

It's overwhelming. And it often shows up right when you have the least amount of energy to deal with it.

Rochelle knows this anxiety well: "We kept getting bills for things I thought were covered. I'd call, be on hold for an hour, get transferred five times, and still have no answers. Every time I opened the mailbox, my chest tightened. It became a source of panic."

For those who aren't familiar with how insurance works (and really, why would you be unless you've had to be?), here's what I've learned: it's complicated on purpose. Systems are designed to save money. And that often means making patients responsible for catching the mistakes. Referrals get lost. Claims are denied. Procedures require prior authorization, even when they're time-sensitive or necessary for your treatment. And while you're trying to manage your health, you're also managing hours of phone calls, stacks of letters, and the emotional toll of trying to advocate for yourself when you're already running on fumes.

Andrea lived that frustration during a moment she'll never forget. "I remember standing in the Walgreens parking lot, crying because my insurance denied my anti-nausea meds. I was puking every hour and they wanted me to try two cheaper options first, even though my oncologist had already said those wouldn't work. It felt like they didn't care if I suffered."

And for Mina, the rules shifted mid-treatment. "Midway through radiation, my insurance changed providers and my deductible reset. Suddenly I owed thousands I wasn't prepared for. I felt like I was being punished for surviving."

We can't always fix the system. But we can talk about it. We can share resources. We can say out loud what too many are suffering through in silence. And sometimes, that acknowledgment, the simple act of being seen, is the first step toward healing, too.

Tips for Taking Back Control

You don't need to become a billing expert overnight. But there are small things that can make a big difference.

Start by creating a folder or binder where you can store everything: bills, Explanation of Benefits (EOBs), letters from insurance, and treatment summaries. Keep a notebook just for phone calls. Write down the name of the person you spoke with, the date and time, and what was said. If they give you a reference or call number, jot that down too.

Always ask for things in writing. If someone tells you something important, like an authorization number or confirmation that a procedure is covered, ask them to send it to you. Get it in writing, and keep a copy.

Follow up. Don't wait on return calls. It's okay to be persistent. You're not being a burden. You're being your own advocate.

And if your hospital has a patient navigator or financial advocate, connect with them. These roles exist to help you. Let them.

Dealing with Bills While You Heal

Cancer is expensive in ways no one really prepares you for. It's not just the chemo drugs or the surgery. It's the scans, the bloodwork, the port flushes. It's the anti-nausea meds that cost more than your car payment, the missed work hours, and the endless appointments, each one carrying its own hidden cost.

And just when you think you've wrapped your head around one charge, another surprise bill shows up. Sometimes months after the fact.

There's no rhythm to it. Bills arrive out of order. Some are duplicates. Some don't even seem related to your care. And yet you're expected to interpret them, track them, and pay them all while your body is still trying to recover.

Write everything down. It doesn't need to be anything fancy. A notebook. A spreadsheet. Even the notes app on your phone. Track when the bill arrived, what it's for, and whether you've followed up.

Before paying anything, take a breath and make a call. Was it submitted to insurance? Was it denied? Is it coded correctly? Mistakes happen often, and sometimes all it takes is one phone call to have something reprocessed or removed.

Always ask for an itemized bill. That single step can save you hundreds. You might find charges for services you never received or procedures that were billed twice. It happens more often than people realize.

And if you're uninsured or underinsured, please know this: you still have options. Most hospitals offer payment plans, especially if you ask before the bill goes to collections. Some will even reduce your balance if you pay a portion up front. Many have financial assistance programs. They just don't always tell you about them unless you ask.

I once heard a story from Ann-Marie, who shared what her sister went through. Her sister felt a lump in November but was between jobs. She waited to get it checked out until her new job's insurance kicked in, but by then, the cancer had metastasized. Tragically, her employer later let her go, likely to avoid the financial burden of her treatment. But Moffitt Cancer Center in Tampa took her in. They covered most of her treatment and gave her a fighting chance.

It was a painful reminder that the system doesn't always make room for the sick. But it was also a reminder that good people and good institutions still exist. You just may have to dig to find them.

💰 Finding Financial Support

The truth is, help exists, but it's often buried under exhaustion, red tape, and forms you don't have the strength to fill out. That's where financial counselors can be a lifeline. Most larger hospitals have someone in this role. Their job is to help patients navigate costs, apply for assistance, and reduce the stress of trying to figure it all out alone.

They can walk you through charity care applications, sliding-scale billing, and programs that quietly forgive medical debt. They know the systems and the shortcuts. And they're often the reason someone gets help they didn't even know was available.

Outside the hospital walls, there's a whole world of organizations built for exactly this. The Pink Fund helps cover everyday expenses like the mortgage, utilities, and car payments, while you're in active treatment. CancerCare offers grants and copay assistance, along with free counseling to support your mental health. The Patient Advocate Foundation connects you with trained case managers who can help fight insurance denials and secure funding for uncovered needs. Triage Cancer provides financial and legal education tailored to the cancer journey.

If prescription costs are overwhelming, check NeedyMeds, GoodRx, or RxAssist. These programs can often slash the cost of life-saving medications and may even connect you directly with pharmaceutical assistance programs.

And if you need to travel for treatment, Hope Lodge, through the American Cancer Society, provides free lodging near major hospitals. Air Charity Network helps with transportation. Even local churches or community organizations may offer gas cards or grocery support. You just have to know where to ask.

The bottom line is this: you don't have to figure it all out alone. Help is out there. And while it may take some effort to access it, every dollar saved, every hour of support gained, is one step closer to peace of mind.

Letting Your Community Step In

When the bills feel insurmountable and your energy is running on fumes, this is where your community can become a lifeline. There is no shame in asking for help. Whether it's financial support, a ride to your appointment, or a warm meal on a hard day, people often want to help. They just need a way to do it.

Crowdfunding platforms like GoFundMe or Facebook Fundraisers give friends, coworkers, and even strangers an avenue to show up for you. Allowing people to step up isn't about pity, but about connection. Shared humanity, and allowing others to participate in your healing.

MealTrain is another powerful tool that lets people sign up to bring meals or deliver groceries without you needing to coordinate a thing. And if even thinking about organizing all this feels too heavy, ask someone you trust to take over the logistics. Appoint a friend or family member to be your communication point. Let them be the one who answers texts, schedules deliveries, and responds to questions.

You didn't ask for cancer. But you can ask for support. Let people love you through it. Let them show up in the ways they can. You are not a burden. You are beloved. And even in your hardest moments, you don't have to walk through it alone.

💼 Disability, Time Off, and Work Options

Cancer doesn't care about timing. It shows up in the middle of work deadlines, parenting duties, and everyday responsibilities. Many people find themselves trying to work through treatment, or navigating a return to work while still physically and emotionally recovering. Whether your employer is supportive or you're left to figure it out alone, understanding your rights and options can make a world of difference.

The Family and Medical Leave Act (FMLA) is one place to start. If you qualify, it offers up to 12 weeks of unpaid, job-protected leave to care for yourself or a loved one. While it doesn't provide income, it does allow you the space to step away from work without fear of losing your job. For those with employer-sponsored benefits, short-term disability may help bridge the gap. It can replace a portion of your income when treatment makes working impossible. And if your recovery takes longer, long-term disability, whether through your employer or a private plan, may continue that support.

If your health prevents you from working indefinitely, Social Security Disability Insurance (SSDI) may be another path to explore. The process is often lengthy and full of documentation, but for many people, it becomes a crucial source of stability. Navigating these programs is not easy, but most cancer centers have social workers or case managers who can guide you through applications, collect the necessary paperwork, and help you understand what's available to you.

If you're nervous about speaking with your employer, it's okay to keep things simple. You can say something like, "I'm undergoing treatment for a medical condition and may need time off or reduced hours. I'm committed to staying in touch and will provide updates as I can." You are not required to explain every detail, and you are absolutely allowed to ask for flexibility. The same strength you bring to your treatment room belongs in your workplace too.

🪙 The Mental Load of Money Stress

When people talk about the financial burden of cancer, they usually mean the bills. But the true weight of it often goes deeper. It's the way your mind loops at night, trying to calculate what's coming and how

274

you'll handle it. It's the tension in your chest when another envelope arrives, and you don't know if it holds an explanation of benefits or a demand for payment. It's the fear of missing something important and the shame that somehow, no matter how hard you try, it still feels like it's not enough.

And then there's the guilt. The guilt of not being able to work or contribute in the same way. The guilt of leaning on friends, on family, on strangers. The guilt of needing help in a world that tells you to handle everything alone. It creeps in quietly, poking holes in your self-worth when you're already trying to hold yourself together.

Denise told me, "I didn't have time to cry. I had work, I had bills, and I had people counting on me. So I showed up to every appointment, took notes, and asked questions. That was how I coped. One task at a time."

There was no room for falling apart. Not because she wasn't scared or overwhelmed but because the rent still needed to be paid, the lights still needed to stay on, and life wasn't going to pause just because cancer showed up.

That kind of strength doesn't always look like peace. Sometimes it looks like spreadsheets and pill organizers and holding back tears in the grocery store. Sometimes it looks like choosing between gas money and prescription co-pays. It's invisible to most people, but it takes everything you've got.

People love to call someone like Denise "strong," but we both know that word doesn't tell the whole story. She did what she had to do to get through it because there wasn't another option. That kind of resilience comes with a price, even if no one sees it.

So let's pause right here and say this clearly: this is not your fault. You are not lazy. You are not irresponsible. You are not a burden. You are a person in crisis trying to survive a broken system. A system that was never designed to support people with compassion. A system that demands strength when you already have nothing left to give.

Your income does not define your value. Your ability to stay caught up on paperwork or make payments on time is not a measure of your worth. You are still you. You are still whole. You are still enough. When that anxiety creeps in and starts to take over, take a breath and remind yourself: "I am not a number on a billing statement."

Then take one small step. Maybe you make one call. Maybe you let someone else open the mail. Maybe all you do today is acknowledge that this is hard, and that you're still doing your best. You were never meant to carry this alone. And you don't have to now.

*Please be sure to review the resources in the back of the book as well! They are there to help you in whatever way they can.

Navigating the Paperwork Maze

Paperwork has a sneaky way of piling up just when you feel least capable of managing it. The stack grows. The language gets more confusing. And the weight of it, both emotional and literal, can start to feel unbearable.

Start small. Make a list of what you know and what you don't. Gather your insurance card, recent bills, explanation of benefits (EOBs), and any letters you've received from your providers. If you're applying for financial assistance, many organizations will ask for documentation about your diagnosis and treatment, recent income, current bills, and sometimes a personal statement or letter from your doctor.

If you're unsure where to begin, reach out to your hospital's financial department. They've seen it all before. And even though it may feel intimidating, remember this: they are there to help you. Bring someone with you if it makes it easier, like a friend, spouse, parent, or trusted advocate. Sometimes just having a second set of ears and an extra set of hands makes all the difference.

And please know this: asking for help isn't a weakness. It's a strategy. It's strength in action. This is exactly why those organizations are there, to help! Every form you fill out, every phone call you make, every question you ask will get you one step closer to your goal.

Even if it doesn't feel like it now, you are doing a brave and powerful thing. And you don't have to do it perfectly. You just need to keep showing up.

✔ Chapter Highlights:

- Insurance and billing issues are common and can feel overwhelming, but they can be managed with organization, persistence, and support.

- Financial support resources exist, including hospital financial counselors, national nonprofits, and local community aid.

- Disability benefits and workplace protections like FMLA can provide stability during and after treatment.

- Money stress affects mental health, and it's okay to ask for help and to let others take over some of the burden.

🩶 Key Takeaway

You didn't ask for cancer, and you certainly didn't ask for the paperwork that comes with it. But even in the middle of chaos, you have the right to clarity, support, and financial peace. Keep asking questions, keep pushing for answers, and let others help you carry the load, because healing shouldn't come with the stress of unpaid bills.

When the load is heavy and the night feels long,
Even small steps forward are brave and strong.
You are not alone in this winding fight
There is help, there is hope, and you hold the light.
— Anonymous

26
Survivorship Guilt & the Comparison Trap

There's a quiet kind of grief that lives inside survival. Most people don't talk about it; not out loud, anyway. It's not quite depression, and it's not the same as mourning someone else. It's more like a shadow that follows you home after the last treatment, waiting in the quiet to whisper, *Why me?*

You ring the bell, hug your nurses, celebrate being "done," and somewhere deep down, you wonder what gives you the right to be okay when others aren't. Maybe it was someone in your support group. Maybe it was the woman who sat next to you in the infusion chair. Even if you barely knew her, her absence hits like a punch to the gut.

Then comes the shame for even feeling that way. People expect you to be grateful, glowing, somehow transformed. But no one warned you about that ache that comes along with surviving. That ache has a name: *survivorship guilt*. And if you've felt it, you are among so many others that have also felt that way.

Cancer rewires the mind. You might find yourself reacting to small moments with big emotions, or pulling away from people who just don't understand. When you try to explain, they tilt their heads and smile, relieved that you're "better," eager for you to move on. But since they have never experienced what you have, they just don't seem to get it. Healing isn't only physical. It's emotional, mental, spiritual. And it doesn't follow the same calendar as your follow-up appointments.

If your thoughts feel messy or too complicated to explain, you're not alone. Many survivors feel the same invisible tug between gratitude and grief.

The Comparison Trap

Amy G. knows that feeling well. "I had a lumpectomy and radiation only," she said. "It's hard sometimes to relate to the breast cancer community, and sometimes I feel like I haven't earned the badge of honor that those who go through chemo have."

That's the comparison trap. The quiet self-doubt that tells you your pain doesn't count because someone else's looks worse. You start to minimize your own story. You wonder if you suffered *enough*. You imagine someone checking your chart and revoking your survivor status.

And then, of course, there's the term some people use: "cancer lite." It's intended as a derogatory remark from those that have undergone surgeries, chemo, and radiation, referring to those that maybe didn't undergo the same experiences. They are basically saying that they had it easier, so their cancer "doesn't count." But there's nothing "lite" about hearing the words *you have cancer*. From that moment on, life changes. You still wake up at 3 a.m. wondering if it will come back. You still hold your breath during every scan. You still carry scars, some seen, some buried deep.

Cancer isn't a contest, and in my mind, there isn't any room for negativity like that. We don't need comparison. We need compassion. Every diagnosis shatters a sense of safety. Every patient walks through fear, hope, and the unknown. Cancer doesn't hand out badges or rank survivors. It just takes, and it changes. There's no hierarchy of pain, and no such thing as "cancer lite."

If you find yourself comparing, pause. Remind yourself: there is no scoreboard. What you went through matters. How you feel matters. You don't need to justify your survival or shrink your story. You've already earned your place at the table.

Where Guilt Comes From

For Melissa B., the guilt came from loss. While she was in treatment for breast cancer, her sister was fighting ovarian cancer and didn't survive. "That has caused some survivor's guilt for me," she shared.

The root of this guilt isn't weakness, it's love. It's the ache of wishing someone else had been given your outcome. It's the human need to find order in the chaos. We tell ourselves that cancer should play by the rules: If you eat well, catch it early, and fight hard, then you'll be okay. But it doesn't always work out that way.

Sometimes cancer takes the young, the kind, the ones who did everything "right." And it spares others without rhyme or reason. So the question shifts from *Why did I get cancer?* to *Why did I get to live?*

That question has no easy answer. But when you recognize guilt as a reflection of love, its grip starts to loosen. You feel guilt because you care deeply. The lives around you matter.

Learning to Carry It

There's no formula for releasing survivor's guilt, but there are gentler ways to hold it. Start by naming it. Let yourself feel it without judgment. Cry, write, sit in silence, or talk it out. Let joy and grief share space, because they can coexist.

You can honor those who didn't make it by living, not by punishing yourself for it. Light a candle, remember their laugh, and let the sunlight in. Talk about them to keep their story alive. But remember that your survival deserves joy too.

When things start to feel too heavy, speak it aloud, to a therapist, a friend, or another survivor who gets it. Saying "I don't know why I'm here and they're not" won't make it worse. It will release some of the pressure. Talking about our problems may not always solve them, but sharing the burden with others makes it easier to carry.

Redefining Survival

Surviving doesn't mean you were stronger or chosen. It means you did.

People might tell you that you have a grand purpose or that God has plans for you, and who knows? Maybe that's true. But maybe your grand purpose is simply to live: to wake up, love deeply, laugh again, and have joy.

As Angela put it, "After I rang the bell, I felt hollow. Everyone was cheering, but I was thinking of the women who didn't make it that far. It didn't feel like a celebration. It felt like betrayal."

Maybe survival is an invitation, not to be perfect, but to be present. To live with softness and boldness. To reach back for someone still caught in the storm.

When the Guilt Softens

At first, guilt hits like a sucker punch. But with time, it softens. It becomes a scar instead of a wound. You'll laugh again and not feel like you're betraying anyone. You'll remember someone you lost and feel warmth instead of pain. You'll cook their favorite meal, play their song, and smile.

You'll realize you didn't survive because you were better or braver. You survived simply because you did. And that's enough.

You're still here writing your story because this life is still yours. Let it be messy, magnificent, and beautiful.

Chapter Highlights

- Survivorship guilt is a painfully personal and often hidden grief that many survivors experience after treatment.

- The comparison trap convinces survivors that their suffering must meet a certain threshold to be valid, but all experiences are worthy.

- Guilt often stems from love and empathy, especially when others did not survive.

- It's okay to hold both joy and grief, and to feel conflicted even during moments of healing.

- Speaking guilt aloud can help loosen its grip and create space for deeper healing.

- Over time, guilt can soften into something quieter, that reminds us of what we've lost while also honoring what we've gained.

🩶 Key Takeaway

You don't have to justify your survival. You don't have to shrink your joy or measure your pain against someone else's. You are allowed to feel thankful and heartbroken at the same time. Guilt doesn't mean you're ungrateful, it means you care for others. And that's something worth honoring.

"Permission"
You are allowed to weep
and still walk in the sun.
To grieve what is lost
and love what's begun.
Healing isn't neat,
nor is it owed—
But every step forward
is a tribute to those
who couldn't.
— Anonymous

27
Moving Forward with Strength & Grace

As I look back on my journey, from a young wife and mother, through a breast cancer diagnosis, a painful divorce, the trials of homelessness, and eventually putting my life back together brick by brick, and then rediscovering love, one truth stands out: resilience is built by making one choice at a time.

In the earliest days, I couldn't imagine offering guidance to someone else. I was barely surviving, one scan, one decision, one breath at a time. I tried to hide from all the trauma behind alcohol and cigarettes, only creating even more trauma. When it comes to cancer, there is no timeline for healing. You don't owe the world your strength before you're ready.

It took me years to reach a place where I could help others without resentment, comparison, or emotional exhaustion. But once I arrived there, I realized something beautiful: giving back has strengthened me. It reminded me of how far I'd come. It gave purpose to my pain.

Don't get me wrong, writing parts of this book took a real toll some days, because I talk about things that happened that I don't normally discuss with other people. Putting it in a book for anybody to ready has been a real challenge, even after all these years. But I feel good knowing that I'm finally at a place where I was ready to share, in hopes that it can help others.

So, whether you're just now finishing treatment or you're years into survivorship, your voice has power. When you're ready, look back, not with bitterness, but with perspective, and ask yourself: "What would I have wanted? Who could I be for someone else?"

You don't have to lead a support group or write a book (though you certainly could). Sometimes, helping looks like sitting next to a newly diagnosed friend and simply saying, "Me too."

There are so many ways to give back, when the time feels right. You might choose to mentor someone who is newly diagnosed, easing their fear and offering them the kind of lived wisdom that no pamphlet or brochure could ever match. Sometimes, being that steady presence can make all the difference. Volunteering at a cancer center or hospital brings connection to patients in active treatment, letting them know they're not alone, even in the hardest moments.

Sharing your story, whether through a blog, a social media post, or standing in front of a room full of strangers, can create ripples of healing. You never know who might see themselves in your journey and feel just a little less alone. Some survivors join patient advisory boards to help shape future care, turning painful lessons into meaningful change for others. Others lend their energy to fundraisers or research events, putting their strength behind innovation and hope.

And sometimes, it's as simple as creating or donating care packages. A soft blanket, a kind note, some lip balm, a tea bag. These small acts say, "Someone sees you."

If you've made it this far, take a moment. Breathe. Acknowledge the weight of what you've just walked through. Not just in these pages, but in your real life. You've gathered information, yes. But more than that, you've given yourself the space to reflect, to feel, and to grow.

You've learned to use your voice in rooms that once felt intimidating. You've reached out, built community, and let yourself be seen. That is not a small thing. Survivorship isn't a finish line. It's not the ribbon at the end of a race. It's a winding, evolving journey that asks you to live fully, love fiercely, and lift others as you go.

There will still be hard days. There will still be moments of doubt or fear. But there will also be joy, connection, and purpose. And now, you have the tools to face all of it with more confidence than before.

Keep leaning on your people: your care team, your loved ones, your fellow survivors. Let them remind you that you are not meant to do this alone.

And most of all, keep going. Set new goals. Take small steps. Let yourself dream bigger than you did before all of this. Celebrate the quiet victories just as much as the big ones. You've made it through so much already. Now, you get to decide what comes next.

May your story be a light for someone still finding their way as you move forward with strength, grace, and grit.

One of the greatest transformations cancer brings has nothing to do with our bodies. It happens quietly inside us, in the way we see the world, in the way we treat people, and in the way we begin to stand up for ourselves, even when our hands still tremble.

For many of us, grace and strength were things we had to learn by fire. Tammy T., diagnosed at 51, shares how her life was cracked wide open by cancer, and how she found meaning, joy, and fierce love in the messy aftermath:

When I look back on my cancer journey, it divides everything, my thoughts, my memories, my life, into two parts: Before Cancer (BC) and After Cancer (AC). There's no returning to the woman I was before that biopsy result popped up on MyChart. I didn't even get the news from my doctor. I opened my phone and saw the word carcinoma, and just like that, the world shifted.

It was our youngest son's first day of 7th grade. I remember exactly where I was. That moment is burned into my brain forever.

I was 51. My kids were 13, 15, and 18. And all I could think was, I have to see them grow up. That was my focus. I knew I had to do everything in my power to stay here for them. That meant a lumpectomy (well, two, to get clear margins), 4 rounds of chemo, 20 rounds of radiation, and now, a mix of Verzenio and aromatase inhibitors for years to come.

I was prepared for the hair loss. I had head wraps and a wig waiting. And yep, right on schedule, I was bald by Thanksgiving. No one ever saw my head uncovered. Not my husband, not my kids, not even my mom. But we still joked about it. My youngest once didn't want to go outside because "the wind would mess up his hair." I looked at him and said, "My hair could blow away, buddy." You either laugh or you cry, and I've done plenty of both.

I kept working through treatment, thanks to an amazing boss and coworkers. I went to my son's basketball game the night after my biopsy and another one just two days after surgery. That's what moms do. We keep showing up, no matter what.

But truthfully, there were days I couldn't hold it together. Days I had to take life one second at a time. I remember one time I was driving alone, and the grief just exploded. I was sobbing and screaming in the car. No audience, no filter, just me, letting it all out. That's how it goes sometimes.

Now that active treatment is over, people assume everything's fine. My hair is growing back (hello, chemo curls), I look "healthy," but I'm still adjusting to this new version of myself. My energy isn't the same. The meds have side effects. The anxiety never really leaves. I still look in the mirror and miss who I used to be. But I'm learning to love the woman I've become.

Every milestone feels bigger now. Watching my kids grow, riding in a monster truck with my oldest, going to a concert, none of it is taken for granted. I laugh at the fact that one of my boobs is firm and perky from radiation, and the other is just along for the ride. That's life now. It's different, but it's mine.

If I could tell someone newly diagnosed one thing, it's this: Take it one step, one breath, one second at a time. You are not alone, even when it feels like it. And when it's hard to believe in your strength, know that there's a whole sisterhood out here who will believe in it for you, until you see it for yourself.

I will never be the same, but I'm still here. And I've got a lot of living left to do.

🐚 The Things People Say

There are moments in the cancer journey when the hardest part isn't the diagnosis, the chemo, or even the pain. Sometimes, it's the way people look at you, or don't. Sometimes, it's the comments they make when they don't realize you're listening. This next piece is my own story, one that reminded me how fragile we can feel and how easily cruelty can cut deep, especially when we're already worn thin.

When I was going through chemo, I lost all my hair, like so many of us do. Living in Florida, it was too hot for wigs or scarves most days, so I often went without. Just me, bald-headed, trying to get through the day.

I was in my early 30s then, and maybe that's why people didn't automatically assume I had cancer. Maybe they thought it was a choice. A fashion statement. Who knows.

One day, I was at the grocery store, walking down an aisle, when I overheard a man in the next row talking to someone. He was talking about me.

Loud enough for me to hear every word, he said he didn't understand why a woman would shave her head. Called it "ugly." He even used the word skinhead.

He wouldn't stop.

I wish I could tell you I confronted him. I wish I had found the words. I wish I'd stood tall and put him in his place.

But I didn't.

I was already feeling broken. Exhausted. Fragile. And in that moment, I didn't have anything left. So I stood there, frozen, letting the words sink in like tiny knives. Each one reminding me how visible and invisible I felt all at once.

That moment has stayed with me, not because I didn't speak up, but because it reminded me how easy it is for people to be cruel without even realizing it. He didn't know I was sick. He didn't know I was barely holding myself together. But that's the point. He didn't need to know. It was none of his business.

You don't need to know someone's story in order to choose kindness. You don't need to understand their full journey to treat them gently. Sometimes the kindest thing you can do is simply stay quiet when you're tempted to judge.

And I wasn't the only one who faced this kind of cruelty. Someone else shared a nearly identical experience:

"I was at Target. A woman with a little girl walked past me, looked me up and down, and whispered, 'Why would anyone choose to look like that?' I didn't even have the energy to respond. I just turned my face away and cried in the shampoo aisle. I wish they knew how much I already missed my hair. How hard it was to look at myself in the mirror."

These encounters leave a mark. But they also teach us what kind of presence we want to be in the world. The example we want to give. After all the opinions, the treatments, and the expectations fade, what we're left with is our own inner landscape. The quiet truths we can no longer ignore. And for many of us, peace doesn't arrive all at once. It finds us in pieces, often in places we least expect.

▽ Finding Peace in Unlikely Places

Not everyone's path looks like mine. Your pain may have come from different directions, or shown up in ways no one else could see. But if you're sitting in the aftermath of cancer, or trauma, or loss, wondering what comes next, I want you to know this:

You're allowed to rebuild something new.

You're allowed to question the life you had before and make space for something better. You're allowed to set new boundaries. To rest without apology. To say no without guilt. You're allowed to live a life that fits the person you've become, not the person you were trying to be before cancer upended everything.

You don't have to make peace with every part of what happened. You don't have to wrap it all up with a pretty bow. You just have to be honest about where you are now.

Peace doesn't always come through closure. Sometimes it comes through clarity. Through walking away. Through starting over. Through choosing softness when it would be easier to armor up again.

▼ Looking Back, Years Later

I know it might sound strange, but after all this time, I've come to see cancer as a gift. Not for what it took from me, but for what it forced me to face.

My first marriage was toxic. I'm not here to point fingers. We were just bad for each other. I married too young. I was impatient. Angry. He had his own flaws. We had separated once before and tried again, mostly for the kids. I spent years trying to figure out how to "make him love me," and I'm sure he tried, in his own way. But I was determined to raise my children in a two-parent home. What I didn't stop to ask was how we were raising them.

There was too much drinking, too much fighting, too many emotional landmines. One day we were fine. The next, we were screaming. But I stayed, because I didn't think I had a choice. I didn't have a career. I bartended a couple nights a week, but I didn't make much. I had no savings. No backup plan. I thought this was it. This was my life.

And then cancer happened.

As brutal as it was, it forced me to hit my own version of rock bottom. I couldn't keep holding everything together. I couldn't keep pretending. I couldn't keep sacrificing myself for a life that was breaking me. Cancer didn't just break my body, it cracked open my whole world. And in that devastation, I found the courage to walk away. To choose something different. To choose me.

Now, to be clear: I don't believe God hands out cancer like some twisted intervention plan. I don't believe everyone who gets sick is supposed to burn their life down and start over. But this was my story. And this is how I've made peace with it.

My daughters have grown into strong, beautiful, emotionally healthy women. And truthfully, I don't know if that would've happened if I had stayed and let then constantly see the fighting.

Linda shared something that stayed with me. "It's been seven years since my last treatment. At first, I held my breath, waiting for the cancer to come back. But over time, something shifted. I stopped waiting for the other shoe to drop and started living again. I still carry the fear sometimes, but it's quieter now. I garden more. I say 'no' more. I look in the mirror and see a woman who fought hard to still be here, and I'm finally proud of her."

And then there was Carmen, who described peace in the most unexpected place. "I didn't think I'd ever stop grieving my old life. But one day, I caught myself singing in the car with the windows down. Just singing. No agenda, no sadness, no fear. And I realized I hadn't thought about cancer in days. It wasn't a big moment. It was a soft one. That's how peace found me. Quietly. In the middle of my ordinary, beautiful, post-cancer life."

This is what I want you to know:
There is life on the other side of this. A good life. A full life.
It won't look the way it used to. But that doesn't mean it won't be beautiful.
Let the light find you in the small things. Let healing come slowly. Let it unfold however it needs to.

You are not finished. You are becoming.

▽ Joyce's Peace Was Already There

Joyce's version of peace looked very different from mine.

She didn't have to rebuild her life after cancer. She didn't need to claw her way toward stability or cut ties to survive. For her, peace came through knowing that what she already had was enough, and that it would still be enough, even if she wasn't there to see it through.

She didn't lie awake wondering if her marriage would survive. Her husband was steady and loving. She didn't question whether her children would be okay. They had already shown her just how strong and capable they were. And when her support system rose up around her like a protective wall of her church family, her coworkers, and her friends, she didn't fight it. She received it with gratitude.

Joyce didn't need to reinvent her life after cancer. She just kept living it. And that in itself was a kind of healing.

When I read her words about trust and about letting go of fear, I realized that peace doesn't always arrive in the aftermath. Sometimes it's been quietly present all along.

✓ Chapter Highlights:

- Survivorship may lead to transformation: new relationships, new boundaries, new ways of living with intention.

- Not everyone's "after" looks the same. Some rebuild. Some rest. Some quietly continue. All of it is valid.

- Giving back, when you're ready, can be genuinely healing, but it's never a requirement.

♥ Key Takeaway

You don't have to return to who you were before cancer. You're allowed to become someone new. Whether you rebuild or simply keep breathing, this life still belongs to you.

"Hope" is the thing with feathers
That perches in the soul
And sings the tune without the words
And never stops
at all
And sweetest
in the Gale
is heard
And sore must be the storm
That could abash the little Bird That kept so many warm
I've heard it in the chillest land
And on the strangest Sea
Yet
never
in Extremity, It asked a crumb
of Me.
— Emily Dickinson

28
Across the Map: Where Healing Finds You

If cancer is a journey, then healing should be too. Not the sterile kind with fluorescent lights and echoing hallways, but something to be experienced with open skies, porch swings, ocean tides, and mountain air. The kind of healing that wraps around your senses, reminds you you're still alive, and gives you permission to be yourself again. After the diagnosis, after the surgery, after the chemo, after the fog, there are places across the country built just for you. Places where we have cried, laughed, let go, and slowly, gently, begun again. You'll find these organizations listed in the back of this book as a resource guide.

When you're deep in the chaos of cancer, it can feel like you're drowning in a checklist. You're trying to stay strong for your family, keep up with doctor's appointments, manage side effects, remember the next prescription, and push through the exhaustion like you've got something to prove. Everyone keeps calling you a warrior, and maybe you've started to believe you have to be one. But you don't. You can take a breath. You can let the mask slip. You can give yourself the grace to just be.

The places you're about to read about can give you that space. They let you take off the armor for a while. Let your body heal without the weight of expectations. Let your mind breathe. And maybe most importantly, they surround you with people who get it. People who've walked the same road, who won't flinch when you talk about drains or panic attacks or the moment you didn't recognize yourself in the mirror. These are places where healing doesn't just happen in your cells, but in your soul.

Let's begin on the coast of Southern California. Here, **Boarding for Breast Cancer (B4BC)** offers surf and wellness retreats that help survivors reconnect with their bodies, the ocean, and each other. Founded by pro snowboarder Megan Pischke, B4BC is also home to the documentary *Chasing Sunshine*, which follows Megan's raw, courageous treatment journey. The women who attend these retreats aren't just learning how to stand on a board, they're learning how to stand back up in life. They paddle into the waves together, laugh when they wipe out, and cry under stars around a fire. It's gritty, healing work disguised as a beach day, and it's so much more powerful than it looks on paper.

Next, in the mountains of Vermont, **Casting for Recovery** invites women to step into waders and into stillness. The rhythm of fly fishing becomes a kind of moving meditation. One survivor said she never thought she'd feel peace again, until she was waist-deep in cold water, casting and crying in the same breath. There's something sacred in that quiet. It makes you slow down. Breathe. And for a little while, it gives your mind and body a place to rest.

Over in North Carolina, **Little Pink Houses of Hope** offers weeklong, beachside retreats for survivors and their families. This isn't just a vacation. It's a way to remember who you are outside of cancer. It's watching your kid belly laugh again, seeing your partner exhale for the first time in months, feeling the wind in your face without the weight of your diagnosis pressing down on you. It's healing through joy, and sometimes joy feels like the most rebellious thing you can choose.

In Tennessee, **Waves of Grace** sends families on oceanfront vacations that are fully funded and filled with soft, beautiful moments. Quiet mornings with coffee on the porch. Holding hands as you walk along the shore. Reading an entire book for the first time in years because no one needs you for anything in that moment. And because they hire photographers, you leave with proof that you did more than survive. You lived.

On the New Jersey shore, **Mary's Place by the Sea** offers a quiet place to fall apart or come back together, whichever you need most. You can spend your time rocking on the porch, eating nourishing meals, or taking deep breaths in a room where no one expects anything from you. It's rest. Real rest. The kind that doesn't come with guilt or pressure.

High up in the Utah mountains, the **Image Reborn Foundation** hosts weekend retreats filled with spa treatments, soul work, and quiet reflection. There are journaling circles lit by candlelight, nature walks that remind you your body can still carry you, and gentle moments that say, "You matter."

If you're looking for something wilder, **First Descents** is your place. This one's for the young adults who want to climb something, paddle something, or scream into the wind. They'll throw you into a kayak or harness and remind you that you are not breakable. You are powerful. You are here.

And finally, if travel isn't an option right now, **Living Beyond Breast Cancer (LBBC)** meets you exactly where you are, whether that's on your couch in pajamas or at 2 AM when the fear won't let you sleep. Their support is quiet, steady, and always there when you need it most.

Cancer may have started this journey. But healing is up to you now. These organizations, listed in the resource section in the back of this book, are scattered across the country like little lighthouses. Go to the ones that call to you. Stand on the shore, climb the mountain, sit on the porch. Wherever healing finds you, let it in.

Chapter Highlights:

- These healing retreats and organizations give you the chance to just *be*. To slow down, breathe, and let go.

- There's something comforting about being surrounded by people who understand without needing explanation.

Key Takeaway

You don't have to go through this alone. There are people and places across the country waiting to meet you exactly where you are, with grace, compassion, and a quiet place to rest. Healing is possible. Connection is powerful. And you are so worthy of both.

"You can't calm the storm... so stop trying. What you can do is calm yourself. The storm will pass."
— Timber Hawkeye

Closing Reflection: A Softer Path Forward

Well, look at you, making it to the end of this book. I don't know whether to hug you or hand you a trophy. Maybe both. Either way, thank you, truly, for walking this road with me. For reading through the messy, the painful, the hopeful, and the absolutely batshit parts of what cancer can do to a life.

We've covered a lot. The sucker punch of diagnosis. The maze of treatment. The scars, the puking, the pity stares. We've tackled the emotional rollercoaster, the identity crisis, the weird-side effects no one warned you about (hello, chemo brain and nipple numbness). We've dragged insurance paperwork through the mud and lit a small, righteous fire under toxic positivity. And still, we made space for softness. For grace. For laughing when it's wildly inappropriate and crying when it's inconvenient.

And through every chapter, every tear-stained memory, every side-eyed moment of "What the actual hell is happening to me?"—my hope was this:
That you felt just a little less alone.
That something here gave you words for what you couldn't quite say out loud.
That you saw yourself in these pages and felt braver for it.

If even one sentence helped you take a deeper breath, or make a hard decision, or simply not throat-punch someone who said, "But you don't look sick," then dragging myself back through all of it to write this book for you was worth it.

Now, I won't bullshit you. I can't promise how your journey will unfold. No one can. Cancer doesn't care about our plans. But I can promise this:
You are stronger than you give yourself credit for.
You are not broken, even when it feels like you've broken in two.
And even on the days when you want to throw your shoe at the wall and just eat cake for breakfast, you are still worthy of love, rest, joy, and ridiculous amounts of hope.

You don't have to be brave all the time. That's a lie the world tells us. You just have to keep going, one stubborn, beautiful, pissed-off, hopeful step at a time.

And if your path looked nothing like mine? If your journey through this mess was gentler. Or messier. Or nothing like what the movies or the pamphlets prepare you for? You're still valid. You don't owe anyone a warrior pose. You don't have to match your pain to someone else's to prove it's real. This book was never about comparison. This book has always been about connection.

Like Nikki, who told me, "Three years out and I finally feel like myself again, except not really. I'm not who I was. I'm softer. Fiercer. I cry more. I laugh louder. I let shit go faster. I don't hustle for anyone's approval anymore. If you don't like me now, that's your loss. I survived hell with a smile and no eyebrows. I'm not here to perform for anyone."

Or Tina, who said, "I used to think survival meant I had to be grateful all the time. But sometimes, I'm just annoyed. My joints hurt. My boobs are uneven. And if one more person tells me how lucky I am, I might scream. But I'm here. And I get to decide how I feel about that. Some days, that's joy. Some days, it's rage. But all of it's real."

This is what life after cancer really looks like. It's not always pretty, but it is immensely personal. You won't just step back into the life you had before. That life doesn't fit anymore. You grow into something else. Someone else. Someone wiser. Someone who survived the fire and carries the smoke in her lungs but still finds a way to sing.

So here's what I'll leave you with:
Take what served you. Leave what didn't.
And carry forward knowing that even if we never meet in person, I'm rooting for you. Hard.

Because you, my friend, are still here. Still standing. Still becoming. And that is a damn miracle.

With love, fire, and a whole lot of
fuck-you-cancer grit,
Brenda M. Lee

📚 Resources for Further Support

This list was created to help you continue learning, healing, and advocating for yourself and your loved ones. Some of these sources guided my own journey. Others were used in the making of this book. Whether you're newly diagnosed, in treatment, rebuilding your life, or supporting someone through it, these resources are here to help.

🩺 Understanding Breast Cancer

American Cancer Society – www.cancer.org
A wide-reaching source for cancer basics, diagnosis explanations, treatment guides, and patient tools.

National Cancer Institute (NCI) – www.cancer.gov
Government-backed site offering detailed, research-based information on all aspects of breast cancer.

BreastCancer.org – www.breastcancer.org
One of the most comprehensive, reader-friendly sites for learning about diagnosis, treatment, types, and side effects.

Susan G. Komen Foundation – www.komen.org
National advocacy organization with information on breast cancer facts, current research, local events, and support programs.

Living Beyond Breast Cancer (LBBC) – www.lbbc.org
A powerful resource throughout every phase—from diagnosis to long-term survivorship. Also offers events, webinars, and a side effects library.

Young Survival Coalition – www.youngsurvival.org
Focused on people diagnosed with breast cancer under age 40, offering peer connection, resources, and advocacy tools.

Metastatic Breast Cancer Network – www.mbcn.org
Educational support and community connection for people living with metastatic breast cancer.

Making Treatment Decisions

NCCN Guidelines for Patients – www.nccn.org/patients
Professional treatment standards in plain language, organized by cancer type and stage.

American Society of Clinical Oncology (ASCO) – www.cancer.net
Research-backed guides on treatment types, side effects, clinical trials, and survivorship.

Radiation Therapy Oncology Group (RTOG) – www.rtog.org
Clinical trial network focused on improving radiation therapy outcomes.

BreastCancer.org – Treatments – www.breastcancer.org/treatment
Explains different treatments, what to expect, and questions to ask your care team.

Cancer.Net – How Cancer Is Treated – www.cancer.net/navigating-cancer-care/how-cancer-is-treated
Helpful breakdowns of surgery, chemo, radiation, targeted therapy, and integrative options.

Support During Care

Cancer Support Community – www.cancersupportcommunity.org
Nationwide network of in-person and virtual support groups, mind-body classes, and education.

Gilda's Club – www.gildasclub.org
Named after comedian Gilda Radner, these clubhouse-style programs offer laughter, learning, and support.

Cancer Hope Network – www.cancerhopenetwork.org
Peer mentorship program connecting newly diagnosed patients with trained volunteers.

CancerCare – www.cancercare.org
Free counseling, support groups, and limited financial assistance for
patients and caregivers.

Look Good Feel Better – www.lookgoodfeelbetter.org
Workshops and tips on skincare, makeup, and self-image during
treatment.

Cancer and Careers – www.cancerandcareers.org
Helps you balance work and cancer treatment, with resources for
employees, employers, and job-seekers.

My Cancer Circle – www.mycancercircle.net
A free tool to coordinate help from family and friends—meals, rides,
errands, and emotional support.

☺ **Fertility & Family Planning After Cancer**

Livestrong Fertility – www.livestrong.org/fertility
Helps patients understand fertility risks and connect with discounted
preservation services.

Oncofertility Consortium – www.oncofertility.northwestern.edu
Educational site offering science-based guidance for patients and
providers.

Alliance for Fertility Preservation –
www.allianceforfertilitypreservation.org
Raises awareness and helps expand access to fertility services.

Motherhood After Cancer – www.motherhoodaftercancer.com
A blog and support space for women navigating parenting during or
after cancer.

RESOLVE: The National Infertility Association – www.resolve.org
Comprehensive resource for people facing fertility issues, including
legal rights and mental health tools.

🪶 Life After Treatment

Dana-Farber – Survivorship Resources – www.dana-farber.org
Includes post-treatment guidelines, emotional support, and long-term follow-up care.

Cancer.Net – Life After Cancer – www.cancer.net/survivorship
Guides on transitioning out of active treatment and what to expect during follow-up.

LBBC – Managing Stress & Anxiety – LBBC Stress & Anxiety Guide (PDF)
Free downloadable guide with calming techniques and emotional coping tools.

Cognitive Rehabilitation After Cancer – Dr. Barbara Collins
A workbook written by a neuropsychologist to help rebuild memory and focus post-chemo.

Insight Timer (App) – www.insighttimer.com
Meditation and relaxation app with free guided sessions for sleep, stress, and focus.

Lumosity – www.lumosity.com
Brain-training games to support memory, speed, and mental flexibility.

Elevate – www.elevateapp.com
Daily cognitive workouts designed to help you feel mentally sharper.

🧠 Mental Health & Emotional Recovery

Psychology Today – www.psychologytoday.com
Find a licensed therapist near you using filters like location, specialty (such as cancer trauma, grief, or anxiety), and insurance coverage. A helpful first step if you're navigating the emotional aftermath of diagnosis or treatment.

Headspace (App) – www.headspace.com
Meditation, mindfulness, and sleep support all in one easy-to-use app.

Some sessions are designed specifically for cancer-related stress, but the broader library is useful for anxiety, restlessness, and mental reset.

💚 Intimacy, Sexual Health & Body Image

WomanLab – www.womanlab.org
Developed by Dr. Stacy Tessler Lindau, WomanLab offers real, research-based answers to questions about intimacy, painful sex, menopause, and body image. It's one of the few places that speaks openly and compassionately about sexual wellness after cancer.

After Cancer – www.aftercancer.co.uk
Though based in the UK, this survivor-led site offers honest stories and tips on self-image, relationships, scars, and reclaiming your identity. A gentle, validating space for long-haul healing.

SHARE: Sexual Health After Cancer – www.sharecancersupport.org
Webinars, Q&As, and articles from a women-led organization focused on often-ignored topics like vaginal dryness, libido changes, and how to talk to your partner about what's different.

Book: "Sex After Cancer" by Dr. Saketh R. Guntupalli & Maryann Karinch
A down-to-earth, empowering guide that breaks the silence around intimacy after treatment. Combines medical expertise with emotional insights and practical suggestions.

🌸 Nutrition, Movement & Wellness

Academy of Nutrition and Dietetics – www.eatright.org
Reliable guidance on diet, nutrition, and survivorship.

Cook for Your Life – www.cookforyourlife.org
Cancer-focused recipes and cooking tips tailored to your needs.

Savor Health – www.savorhealth.com
Offers AI-powered meal plans and nutrition support.

Blue Zones Project – www.bluezones.com
Healthy living strategies based on the world's longest-living
populations.

National Center for Complementary & Integrative Health –
www.nccih.nih.gov
Science-based info on herbs, supplements, and alternative healing.

Yoga4Cancer (y4c) – www.yoga4cancer.com
Certified yoga program specifically designed for cancer patients and
survivors.

Moving Through Cancer – Dr. Kathryn Schmitz –
www.movingthroughcancer.com
Exercise-based cancer recovery program by a leading researcher.

Dana-Farber – Post-Mastectomy Exercises – www.dana-farber.org
Illustrated PDF for post-surgical healing and mobility.

LympheDIVAs – www.lymphedivas.com
Stylish compression garments and education for managing
lymphedema.

🎗 Financial & Legal Help

Cancer Financial Assistance Coalition (CFAC) – www.cancerfac.org
Searchable database of national and regional financial aid programs.

Triage Cancer – www.triagecancer.org
Free education on legal and insurance rights for cancer patients.

NeedyMeds – www.needymeds.org
Find discounts on prescriptions, medical services, and transportation.

Patient Advocate Foundation – Co-Pay Relief – www.copays.org
Financial assistance for copays, premiums, and treatment costs.

HealthWell Foundation – www.healthwellfoundation.org
Helps cover out-of-pocket expenses for people with serious diseases.

Family Reach – www.familyreach.org
Provides grants for living expenses like rent and food during treatment.

The Pink Fund – www.pinkfund.org
Short-term financial help for people in active treatment.

United Way 211 – www.211.org
Call 211 or search online to connect with local support services.

The Assistance Fund – www.tafcares.org
Supports underinsured patients with out-of-pocket medical costs.

Good Days – www.mygooddays.org
Helps people afford life-saving and life-extending medications.

Healing, Spirituality & Integrative Care

HealingStrong – www.healingstrong.org
Faith-based cancer support groups focused on natural healing.

Society for Integrative Oncology – www.integrativeonc.org
Evidence-based practices combining traditional and holistic care.

Find a Naturopathic Doctor – www.naturopathic.org
Directory of licensed naturopathic physicians by region.

Find an Acupuncturist (NCCAOM) – www.nccaom.org
Search for certified practitioners of Chinese medicine and acupuncture.

Memorial Sloan Kettering – About Herbs – www.mskcc.org/herbs
Evidence-based resource on herbal supplements and interactions.

Center for Mind-Body Medicine – www.cmbm.org
Mindfulness, trauma recovery, and integrative self-healing programs.

🧬 Special Populations

The National LGBT Cancer Network – www.cancer-network.org
Provides culturally competent care resources, support groups, and
advocacy for LGBTQIA+ cancer patients and survivors.

FORCE LGBTQ+ Community – www.facingourrisk.org
A dedicated part of the FORCE network that addresses hereditary
cancer risk and advocacy with LGBTQ+ individuals in mind.

Stupid Cancer – www.stupidcancer.org
Support and events for adolescent and young adult (AYA) cancer
patients.

Elephants and Tea – www.elephantsandtea.org
Platform for AYA patients to share stories and connect.

The Samfund – www.thesamfund.org
Financial grants for young adults rebuilding after cancer.

Male Breast Cancer Coalition – www.malebreastcancercoalition.org
Awareness and support for men with breast cancer.

Young Men's Breast Cancer Support – www.youngmensbc.org
Resources tailored to men diagnosed under age 50.

FORCE: Facing Our Risk of Cancer Empowered –
www.facingourrisk.org
Education and advocacy for hereditary cancers like BRCA.

National Society of Genetic Counselors – www.nsgc.org
Helps you locate genetic counselors for hereditary risk questions.

👥 Caregivers & Partners

CaringBridge – www.caringbridge.org
A free and private space to keep family and friends updated during

treatment. Caregivers can use it to coordinate support, share medical updates, and reduce the emotional labor of repeating information.

Well Spouse Association – www.wellspouse.org
Offers connection, validation, and practical support for spouses and partners who have become long-term caregivers. A powerful reminder that you're not alone in this role.

Family Caregiver Alliance – www.caregiver.org
Education, legal tools, and emotional support tailored for unpaid caregivers navigating the complexities of cancer care. Includes a state-by-state guide to local programs.

💔 Grief, Loss & End-of-Life Support

GriefShare – www.griefshare.org
In-person and online grief support groups led by trained facilitators.

The Dougy Center – www.dougy.org
Specializes in bereavement support for children and teens.

What's Your Grief – www.whatsyourgrief.com
Coping tools, articles, and courses for all types of grief.

Hospice Foundation of America – www.hospicefoundation.org
Grief education, caregiving tools, and end-of-life resources.

National Alliance for Children's Grief – www.childrengrieve.org
Resources for families and professionals supporting grieving children.

📋 Crisis Support & Connection

988 Suicide & Crisis Lifeline – www.988lifeline.org
Call or text 988 anytime for immediate emotional support.

Veterans Crisis Line – www.veteranscrisisline.net
Support for veterans in crisis. Call 988 and press 1.

Crisis Text Line – Text HOME to 741741
Confidential, 24/7 text support from trained counselors.

National Domestic Violence Hotline – www.thehotline.org
Support, safety planning, and resources. Call 1-800-799-SAFE.

Samaritans (International) – www.samaritans.org
Global crisis line with support in multiple languages.

Reddit: r/breastcancer – www.reddit.com/r/breastcancer
A peer-support forum for sharing stories and advice.

Facebook Support Groups – Search: Breast Cancer Support Network,
Thrivers Club, Young Survivors Unite
Real-time connection and shared experience in private group settings.

Relay for Life (ACS) – secure.acsevents.org
Community events honoring survivors and raising funds.

Living Beyond Breast Cancer – Resource Hub – www.lbbc.org/
community/breast-cancer-resources A comprehensive directory of
articles, videos, and support tools.

🏕 **Healing Retreats & Reconnection**

Boarding for Breast Cancer (B4BC) – www.b4bc.org
Surf and wellness retreats, survivor meetups, and educational resources.

Casting for Recovery – www.castingforrecovery.org
Free fly-fishing retreats for breast cancer survivors across the U.S.

Little Pink Houses of Hope – www.littlepink.org
Week-long beach retreats for breast cancer patients and families.

Waves of Grace – www.waves-of-grace.org
Free coastal vacations for families facing cancer, including
photography services.

Mary's Place by the Sea – www.marysplacebythesea.org
Holistic healing and rest for women with cancer in a peaceful
shorefront home.

Image Reborn Foundation – www.imagerebornfoundation.org
Weekend retreats in Utah for women recovering from breast cancer.

First Descents – www.firstdescents.org
Outdoor adventure programs for young adults impacted by cancer.

Living Beyond Breast Cancer (LBBC) – www.lbbc.org
Also offers in-person conferences and virtual healing sessions.

📖 Voices, Stories & Survivor-Led Healing

Because sometimes what we need most isn't another medical article—
it's a voice that sounds like ours. These podcasts and books are created
by, for, and about people navigating life with and after breast cancer.
They're raw, real, and deeply human.

🎧 *The Cancer Mavericks* **(by GRYT Health)**
A storytelling podcast featuring patients and survivors who challenged
the system—and changed it. Moving, powerful, and full of heart.

🎧 *Breast Cancer Stories*
One woman's breast cancer journey, told in real time. From discovery
through reconstruction, this podcast offers a brave, unfiltered look into
what so many of us go through behind closed doors.

📖 *Sex After Cancer* **by Dr. Saketh R. Guntupalli & Maryann Karinch**
A must-read for anyone struggling with intimacy, self-image, or
reconnection post-treatment. Equal parts compassionate and practical.

About the Author

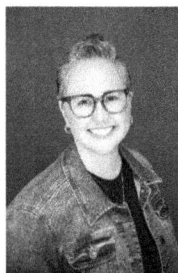

Brenda M. Lee is a U.S. Navy veteran, writer, and photographer who brings compassion, grit, and vulnerability to every story she tells. As the first female parachute rigger assigned to a seagoing squadron, with orders approved by Congress, Brenda broke barriers for women in the military while serving her country, and later faced one of life's hardest battles: breast cancer.

Born and raised on a farm in Michigan, she now lives in Green Cove Springs, Florida, where she continues her creative work through photography and passion projects. While Brenda's professional life has spanned aircraft maintenance, owning a bakery, learning photography, and artistic storytelling, her most important roles have been those of mother, bonus-mother, and grandmother to a beautifully blended family, whom she lovingly describes as "collected."

Seventeen years after beating breast cancer, and just a month before turning fifty, Brenda gave back in an extraordinary way: she donated a kidney to a close family member. It was a powerful reminder that healing can come full circle, and that strength built through survival can one day save another life.

Her experience with breast cancer, along with the emotional, physical, and relational toll it took, led her to write this book not as a medical guide, but as a personal companion for others walking the same path. She hopes her words offer comfort, perspective, and strength to those facing their own diagnosis.

"This book was born from my story, but it's for yours. Please share it. Someone you love may need these pages more than you know."

To learn more about Brenda or subscribe to her blog, visit

https://brendamlee.wordpress.com/